Basic Psychology for Nurses

Basic Psychology for Nurses

(As per INC Syllabus)

Rajesh Kumar MSc (N) PhD
Assistant Professor
College of Nursing
All India Institute of Medical Sciences (AIIMS)
Rishikesh, Uttarakhand, India

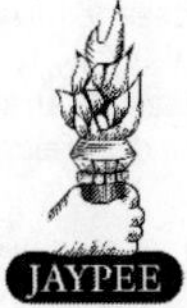

JAYPEE BROTHERS MEDICAL PUBLISHERS
The Health Sciences Publisher
New Delhi | London

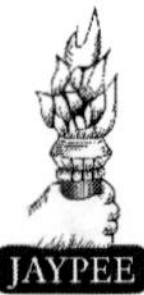

JAYPEE **Jaypee Brothers Medical Publishers (P) Ltd**

Headquarters
EMCA House
23/23-B, Ansari Road, Daryaganj
New Delhi 110 002, India
Landline: +91-11-23272143, +91-11-23272703
+91-11-23282021, +91-11-23245672
E-mail: jaypee@jaypeebrothers.com

Corporate Office
4838/24, Ansari Road, Daryaganj
New Delhi 110 002, India
Phone: +91-11-43574357
Fax: +91-11-43574314
E-mail: jaypee@jaypeebrothers.com

Overseas Office
J.P. Medical Ltd
83 Victoria Street, London
SW1H 0HW (UK)
Phone: +44 20 3170 8910
E-mail: info@jpmedpub.com

EU GPSR Authorised Representative
Logos Europe, 9 rue Nicolas Poussin
17000, La Rochelle, France
Phone: +33 (0) 6 67 93 73 78
E-mail: contact@logoseurope.eu

Website: www.jaypeebrothers.com
Website: www.jaypeedigital.com

Inquiries for bulk sales may be solicited at: jaypee@jaypeebrothers.com

Basic Psychology for Nurses

First Edition: 2018

Reprint: 2025**, 2026**

ISBN: 978-93-5270-216-9

Printed at: Samrat Offset Pvt. Ltd.

Dedication

*I wish to dedicate this book to my beloved mother
who departed from this world just few weeks ago.
Thank you mom for being a symbol of hardwork,
inspiration and dedication in my eyes.
I could not dream my success without
your unconditional love you shower on me!*

Contributors

Achla Dagdu Gaikwad
Associate Professor
Amity College of Nursing
Amity University
Gurgaon, Haryana, India

Aashish Parihar
Lecturer
College of Nursing
AIIMS
Jodhpur, Rajasthan, India

Babita Singh
Associate Professor cum
Vice-Principal
National Medical College and
Nursing Campus
Birgunj, Nepal

Manjula V
Clinical Psychologist
PhD Scholar
Family Therapy Unit
NIMHANS
Bengaluru, Karnataka, India

Raminder Kalra
Principal
Holy Family College of Nursing
New Delhi, India

Sumity Arora Tarafdar
Assistant Professor
Holy Family College of Nursing
New Delhi, India

Sushil K Maheswari
Associate Professor
University College of Nursing
Baba Farid University of
Health Sciences
Faridkot, Punjab, India

Xavier Belsiyal C
Assistant Professor
College of Nursing
AIIMS
Rishikesh, Uttarakhand, India

Preface

Psychology is the scientific study of human behavior which is a complex phenomenon and all are interested to know about common mental process. The study of psychology provides invaluable understanding and develops positive perception about self and other human being.

In spite of availability of a bulk of books and literature, I have written this book keeping in mind the interest of the graduate nursing students.

In my teaching career, I have realized the needs and problem faced by nursing students in examination. Therefore, a modest attempt has been taken to furnish all the possible content as suggested by Indian Nursing Council for BSc and Post Basic BSc nursing students. A simplified and user-friendly approach has been taken care to make the things more understandable and realistic for the nursing students.

This book contains multiple choice questions, short and long answer and essay questions at the end of each chapter. Readymade availability of multiple choice questions, short and long essay questions will help the students in quick review and preparation for final examination. I hope that this book will help fast as well slow learners to understand certain intricate concepts of psychology.

Rajesh Kumar

Acknowledgments

This book is the result of many helping hands, which came in the shape of advisors, colleagues, teachers, family members and many other people. I am thankful to all the contributors from the core of my heart for helping me in completing the task within appropriate time limit.

I would like to acknowledge the comments of reviewers whose feedback greatly influenced me to shape this book. Several of the comments triggered my work and motivated me to refine the content time to time.

Indeed, my humble gratitude and words of appreciation to all the contributors for their timely needed support to bring the book in final shape.

I thank my parents and my wife (*Capt Kalpana*, Ex-Indian Army Officer) and my sweet daughter (*Pihoo*) for showing high degree of patience and sacrifices during the work.

My sincere thanks to the staff of Jaypee Brothers Medical Publishers (P) Ltd, New Delhi for giving me an opportunity to share the knowledge with this book.

Above all, I express my deep sense of gratitude to Lord Almighty for abiding grace and blessings which gave me strength for completing this project successfully.

INC Syllabus

PSYCHOLOGY

Course description: This course is designed to assist the students to acquire knowledge of fundamentals of psychology and develop an insight into behavior of self and others. Further, it is aimed at helping them to practice the principles of mental hygiene for promoting mental health in nursing factors.

Unit No.	Time (hrs)	Learning Objectives	Content	Chapter
I	2	Describe the history, scope and methods of psychology.	**Introduction** • History and origin of science of psychology • Definitions and Scope of psychology • Methods of psychology • Relevance to nursing	1
II	4	Explain the biology of human behavior.	**Biology of behavior** • Body mind relationship modulation process in health and illness • **Genetics and behavior:** Heredity and environment • **Brain and behavior:** Nervous System, Neurons and synapse, • Association Cortex, Rt and Lt Hemispheres • Psychology of Sensations • Muscular and glandular controls of behavior • Nature of behavior of an organism/ Integrated responses	2
III	20	Describe various cognitive processes and their applications.	**Cognitive Processes** • **Attention:** Types, determinants, Duration and degree and alterations • **Perception:** Meaning, Principles, factors affecting and Errors,	3, 4, 5, 6, 7

Unit No.	Time (hrs)	Learning Objectives	Content	Chapter
			• **Learning:** Nature, Types, Learner and learning, Factors influencing, laws and theories, process, transfer and study habits • **Memory:** Meaning, Types, Nature, Factors influencing, Development theories and methods of memorizing and forgetting • **Thinking:** Types and levels, stages of development, Relationship with language and communication • **Intelligence:** Meaning, classification, uses and theories • **Aptitude:** Concept, types, Individual differences and variability • Psychometric assessment of cognitive processes • Alterations in cognitive process • Applications	
IV	8	Describe motivation, emotions, stress, attitudes and their influence on behavior.	**Motivation and Emotional processes** • **Motivation:** Meaning, Concepts, Types, Theories, Motives and behavior, Conflicts and frustration and conflict resolution • Emotions and stress – **Emotion:** Definition, components, Changes in emotions, theories, emotional adjustment, emotions in health and illness – **Stress:** Stressors, cycle, effect, adaptation and coping • **Attitude:** Meaning, nature, development and factors affecting, – Behavior and attitudes – Attitudinal changes • Psychometric assessments of emotions and attitudes • Alterations in emotions • Applications	8, 9, 10

Unit No.	Time (hrs)	Learning Objectives	Content	Chapter
V	7	Explain the concepts of personality and its influence on behavior.	**Personality** • Definitions, topography, types and theories • Psychometric assessments of personality • Personality assessment: objective test, projective test/subjective test. • Alternations in personality • Nursing applications	11
VI	4	Explain the psychological assessment and role of nurse.	**Psychological assessment and tests** • Types of psychological tests • Characteristics of good psychological tests • Uses of psychological tests • Role of nurses in psychological assessment	16
VII	7	Describe psychology of people during the life cycle.	**Developmental Psychology:** • Psychology of people at different ages from infancy to old age • Psychological needs of vulnerable population • Psychology of vulnerable individuals- challenged, women, sick etc • Psychology of groups • Nursing implications	12
VIII	8	Describe the characteristic of mentally healthy person. Explain ego defense mechanisms.	**Mental hygiene and mental Health** • Concepts of mental hygiene and mental health • Characteristics of mentally healthy person • Warning signs of poor mental health • Promotive and preventive mental health- strategies and services • Ego Defense mechanisms and implications • Personal and social adjustments • Guidance and counseling • Role of nurse	13

Contents

Introduction to Psychology

Chapter 1

INTRODUCTION

Human behavior is a complex phenomenon. All are interested in understanding human behavior. Primarily, it was the philosophers who took up the subject of human behavior and tried to find out the cause for such behavior. Thus, psychology has rich roots dating back into philosophy and physiology. Later on, as the element of speculative thinking decreased and objective experimental investigation increased, it gradually developed into a positive science. Now, it has been regarded as an independent branch of study. It explains the recent opening of the independent department of psychology in the various universities. It is the subject of modern era concerned with the study of human being and psychological process that can understand human being in a better way.

Meaning and Definition

Psychology as science of soul: Psychology has come from the Greek word '*psyche*' which means '*soul*' and '*logos*' which means '*to study*'. Thus, psychology means *study of soul.* Hence, it was regarded as a talk about soul. Later on, it was observed that it is better to call psychology as the 'science of soul' rather than to 'talk about soul', as psychology is a science and better word because of the following reasons:

- Science is more systematic and exhaustive than talk. Talk goes on carelessly and loosely. It is usually muddled, vague, indefinite and fragmentary.
- Science is based on practical knowledge and implies it to help in prediction.
- Science helps to improve knowledge based on empirical observation.
- Science uses special technical terminology.

But the definition of considering psychology as study of soul was rejected because of following reasons:

- Nature, origin and place of soul are not known. It has no physical existence, it cannot be seen and heard, it has no height and volume. It is a metaphysical concept.
- It is a theological concept based on certain theories of religion and relationship to god that makes psychology more of religion than a science.
- Soul makes the science speculative as it cannot be verified.

So, the definition of psychology as study of science was unscientific and hence this is discarded.

Psychology as science of mind: The term mind was considered better and it was substituted for soul. Hence, the study of soul psychology changed to the study of mind. Various views about mind:

Laymen's view; mind is something in the body or heart which feels or acts. If mind means something mysterious to ourself it would be just the same as soul. Hence this definition again got rejected.

Psychologist's view; mind is combination of some total of mental process and it stands for personal experiences of man, i.e. pleasure, pain, wishes, hope expectation, dream and desire, etc.

Many other characteristics and mental processes were also explained before rejecting the definition of psychology as study of mind like continuity, unity, immaterial and private.

Criticism of Definition

- Mind is subjective. We can know our own mind but not the others. So it is half true.
- Mind implies continuity and unity but it is lacking in abnormal human being, theories and animals.

Psychology as science of consciousness: Since 1857, psychology was defined as 'science of consciousness'. Consciousness refers to awareness to self and others. Hence, consciousness stands for inner experience of man–his thoughts, feelings and memories, etc.

This definition of psychology as study of mind or consciousness is got rejected due to following reasons:

- A small portion of mind (around 1/10 part) is conscious and remaining most important is unconscious and subconscious and this definition excludes both important areas of mind.

- A human can be conscious to his/her own mental activities and cannot know the consciousness of others. This method is like to introspection which is most subjective and least scientific method.

'Psychology as a science of immediate experience with consciousness being the main subject matter' (Wilhelm Wundt, 1832–1920)

'Psychology is the science of conscious experience which is dependent upon the experiencing person' (Titchner, 1876-1927)

Psychology as science of behavior: This is the most accepted definition of psychology in modern era. Behavior according to Woodworth is a collective nature of various types of activities: cognitive, conative and affective corresponding to knowing, doing and feeling. Behavior is classified in the following three categories:

1. ***Cognitive behavior***: It is concerned with knowing and thinking aspects, e.g. problem-solving
2. ***Affective behavior***: It is concerned with feelings, e.g. anger, fear, jealousy, etc.
3. ***Conative behavior***: It is concerned with motor activity, e.g. cycling, playing and running, etc.

It should be noted that no piece of behavior is purely of one category. It may be having dominance of any one aspects or equal partnership of all three.

Psychology as science of behavior has been defined by various Psychologists, some of these definitions are given below:

'Psychology is a positive science of behavior' (Watson)

'Psychology is a science of behavior and experience' (Skinner)

'Psychology is concerned with the scientific investigation of behavior'

(Munn) 'Psychology is the study of human behavior and human relationship' (Crow and Crow)

'Psychology is concerned with observable human behavior' (Garrison and Others)

Analysis of Definition

If we analyze the definition of psychology given by different psychologists, we shall come to the following conclusions:

- Psychology is regarded as a science.
- It is a positive and empirical science.

- It is a branch of natural science. It is a science of behavior and not of matter. It cannot be called pure science like mathematics and chemistry.
- It studies physical, mental, emotional, and social behavior. It studies cognitive activities like memory, thinking, imagination, learning, intelligence as well as psychophysiological characteristics of the individual.
- It studies the behavior of human being and animals.

Psychology as a Science

In the words of Prof Woodworth, 'psychology can be defined as the science of the activities of the individual in relation to environment'. Let us understand this definition by explaining the various technical terms to justify psychology as a science.

Science–psychology is a science. Science is the systematic and methodological study of any breach of knowledge. A study cannot be called as science merely on the basis of its subject matter; what is even more important is the scientific method. It is the method which is science, not the subject matter. Thus, a characteristics feature of science is its method rather than its field of study. Salient features of science are as follows:

Scientific Method

- A science follows scientific method. The main steps of the scientific method are given below:
  - ***Observation:*** Minute and detailed observation is the first step in scientific method. An observer should use best reliable and valid instrument for observation. The accuracy of the instruments should be ascertained before its use.
  - ***Recording***: The observation should be carefully recorded and reported in its complete manner.
  - ***Classification of findings:*** After recording and writing of observation, the findings collected must be classified and organized in logical sequence.
  - ***Analysis, interpretation and generalization***: The scientific method analyzes the findings and makes them meaningful and generalized to other population. It should be kept in mind that while making generalization some general conclusion is drawn. These generalizations sometimes known as *universal laws*.

- *Verification*: This is the last step in the scientific method. It deals with verification of universal law in order to ascertain their validity. It helps to make the law scientific and universally accepted.

- **Factuality:** Science is the study of facts and figures and the search for true facts.
- **Universality:** Scientific laws are verified and universally accepted.
- **Validity:** Scientific laws are valid at all times and at all places across the globe. They are open to examination at all times. They will be found universally accepted.
- **Discovery of cause and effect relationship:** Science studies cause and effect relationship. It searches for cause and effect relationship.
- **Prediction:** Science makes prediction for future outcome.

So, on the basis of above listed criteria of science, it can be concluded that psychology is a science because;

- Psychology follows scientific method to observe and record the behavior and clarify, analyze, generalized and verified for truth.
- Psychology is based on true facts (empirical and factual).
- Principles of psychology are valid and universally accepted.
- Psychology defines cause and effect relationship.
- Psychology enables to predict.

It should be noted that psychology is a positive empirical science. It is positive because it is concerned with mind and behavior as they actually are. It is empirical because, like other sciences, it uses the method of observation of facts.

Activities

The second technical term used in Woodworth definition was activities. Psychology studies the activities of the individual. The word activity is used here in a very broad sense. In the word of Woodworth, 'any manifestation of life can be called activities'. It includes;

- Physical or motor activities—for example, walking, cycling, playing, boxing, driving and washing, etc.
- Mental or intellectual activities—for example, learning, thinking, remembering, learning and observing, etc.
- Emotional activities—for examples: laughing, crying, smiling, shouting, happy, sad and feeling angry, etc.

Sometimes, these above mentioned activities are classified under three kinds of behavior, i.e. cognitive, conative and affective.

Individual

Psychology is the science of activities of the individual. Individual is a psychophysical organism (having mind and body). Psychology studies activities of all types of individuals, i.e. children, adolescents, adults, normal person, abnormal person, intelligent person, feeble minded person and even animals.

Environment

Psychology studies the activities of individual in relation to the environment. Environment refers to all types of circumstances that influence the behavior of an organism since conception to death. Environment may be physical, intellectual, social, moral, economic and political and cultural forces. All these forces have the influence on the activities, behavior and personality of the individual.

- ***Physical environment:*** It includes food, temperature, climate, home and social building, etc
- ***Intellectual/mental environment***: It consists of books, libraries, laboratories, museum, intellectual takes and interest of parents etc.
- ***Social environment***: It includes members of the family, like parents, relatives, friends and teachers.
- ***Emotional environment***: It consists of emotional nature of family, friends, relatives and teachers.
- ***Relationship*:** It is also noted that there could be three different types of relationship between individual and environment.
  - ***Dependence***: The individual has to depend on environment for the development of emotional, physical, mental and other types of activities and influenced by the way he participates in the environment. His participation influences his environment.
  - ***Participation*:** Individual's physical, social, emotional and mental development is influenced by the way he participates in the environment.
  - ***Interaction*:** The interaction naturally takes place between individual and environment and both affect each other.

So, Psychology can be described as study of the individual which deals with behavior and experience. Individual may be human being or animal, child, adolescent, adult, men, women, normal, gifted, backwards, intelligent, dull and feeble minded, behavior can be good or bad, desirable or undesirable, moral or immoral, sociable or unsociable, it becomes the subject matter of psychology.

BRANCHES AND FIELD OF PSYCHOLOGY (APPLICATION OF PSYCHOLOGY)

The entire study and scope of psychology has been divided in the following branches and fields:

- Normal and abnormal psychology
  - ***Normal psychology***: It studies the behavior and mental processes of normal as well as of abnormal persons. Normal psychology deals with the behavior and mental processes of normal individuals.
  - ***Abnormal psychology***: Abnormal psychology studies the behavior of a person suffering from mental diseases. It studies cause, nature, and preventive measures of abnormal behavior each as hysteria, and phenomena of split personality. Attempts are made to cure abnormal behavior.
- Human and animal psychology
  - ***Human psychology***: It studies the behavior of human being only. Some of the branches of human psychology are described here as follows:
    - ***Child psychology***: It studies physical, motor, intellectual, emotional, social, moral and aesthetic development of the child. It studies the behavior of the child as well as his various aspects of the personality.
    - ***Adolescent psychology***: Adolescents are those people who are in the age group 12 to 19 years. Adolescent psychology deals with behavior and personality pattern of adolescents.
    - ***Adult psychology***: It deals with the behavior of adult human being whose mental level is higher and behavior is more natural than those of children.
  - ***Animal psychology***: Animal psychology studies the behavior of animals. Sometimes it is called comparative psychology because it also compares human behavior to animal behavior. Animal psychology is useful for understanding the human behavior as well.

- Individual and social psychology
  - ***Individual psychology (differential psychology)*:** Individual psychology studies the facts of variations existing among different individuals. Individual differ in respect to physique, intelligence, attitude, achievement, aptitudes, interest, education, race and culture, etc.
  - ***Social psychology (group psychology)***: Social psychology studies the behavior of the individual in relation to social situation. It deals with various types of group phenomena such as public opinion, crowd, propaganda, attitudes, belief, inter-group, inter-race, international conflict and tension. This social psychology studies individual as a member of social group.
- Pure and applied psychology
  - ***Pure psychology*:** When any science is studied for sake of advancement of knowledge, we call it a pure science. But when its study is done with a view to find new knowledge for practical human purposes or social utility, we call it applied sciences. Hence, pure psychology studies the mental processes and behavior of human being and animals to discover fundamental laws and principles underlying their functioning.
  - ***Applied psychology***: Applied psychology applies the general principles of psychology for practical utilities. Some of the branches of applied psychology are described here as follows:
    - ***Legal or criminal psychology*:** Legal or criminal psychology studies the behavior or person with criminal intimidation and various legal proceeding against them.
    - ***Industrial psychology or organizational behavior*:** Industrial psychology studies the industrial problem with regards to selection, placement, efficiency and need of counseling, etc.
    - ***Military psychology*:** This branch deals with the use of psychological principles and techniques in the world of military science; how to keep the morale high during war, how to fight the war of propaganda and intelligence services, how to secure better recruitment of the personal for armed forces and how to improve motivational climate and leadership.

- ***Political psychology:*** This branch relates itself with the use of psychological principles and techniques in studying politics and deriving political games. The knowledge of the dynamic of group behavior, the judgment of public opinion, qualities of leadership, psychology of propaganda and suggested the art of diplomacy are the key concepts of this branch.
- ***Environmental psychology:*** This branch studies how the behavior is influenced by environmental factors such as home, school, space and noise etc. It is proved by various studies that there is a close relationship between environment and behaviors.
- ***Educational psychology:*** This branch tries to apply the psychological principles, theories, and techniques to human behavior in educational situation. The subject matter of this branch is teaching learning process, learning situation, learning material and method, learning environment and teachers.

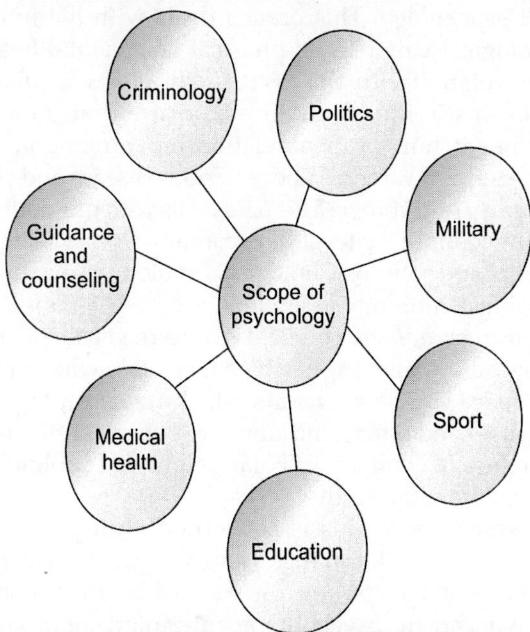

Fig. 1.1: Scope of psychology

- *Clinical psychology:* It describes and explains causes and treatment modalities of abnormal behavior or any kind of mental problem. It suggests psychotherapeutic treatment for people who suffer from mental illness. Psychotherapeutic treatments are psychotherapy, relaxation therapy, cognitive therapy, behavior therapy, family therapy, family drama, etc.
- *Animal psychology:* Animal psychology is concerned with the study of animal behavior under controlled conditions. It deals with the study of animal behavior through various experiment and observations.
- *Developmental psychology:* The subject matter of development psychology is product and process of growth and development of human being from conception till date, various physical and psychological changes, development of personality traits, and other Developmental changes.

Apart from the above listed branches, some emerging trends of psychology are:

- *Health psychology*: This branch deals with the influence of psychological variables as physical and mental health. This field is related with the issue such as stress, depression, psychosomatic illness etc. It also concentrates on hospital environment, nurse patient relationship, promotion of mental health, lack of awareness about various disease and problems.
- *Community psychology*: This field deals with promoting mental health at community level. The community psychologist tries to prevent and solve psychological problems by evaluating and improving community as a whole.
- *Aerospace psychology*: This field is concerned with physiological and psychological changes which take place when individuals are in space crafts or aircrafts which travel on high altitude atmosphere and other conditions are entirely different when a person goes beyond a particular height and prolongs his/her stay away from the earth.
- *Sport psychology*: This is concerned with play and sport activities of human life. It tries to answer questions like what are the motives of players, how can we increase their motivational levels, what are the psychotherapeutic interventions we can do in the field of sports and games.

- ***Physiological psychology***: It is concerned with structure and functions of sense organ, nervous system, glands and muscle underlying our behavior.
- ***Experimental psychology***: It studies mental process and behaviors by means of scientific experiments; mainly in laboratory or controlled condition.
- ***Parapsychology***: It is one of the recent developments of psychology. It deals with problems like extrasensory perception, and telepathy etc. An institute of parapsychology is established in Rajasthan (Sri Ganganagar).
- ***Criminal psychology***: Studying criminal psychology improves the ways and means of crime detection, intentions of criminal person, ways and kind of doing crimes and others related phenomena related to crime.
- ***Geriatric psychology***: It studies various changes in behavior during old age stage, i.e. changes in mood, isolation, feeling of love, sympathy, affection and sexual desire, etc.

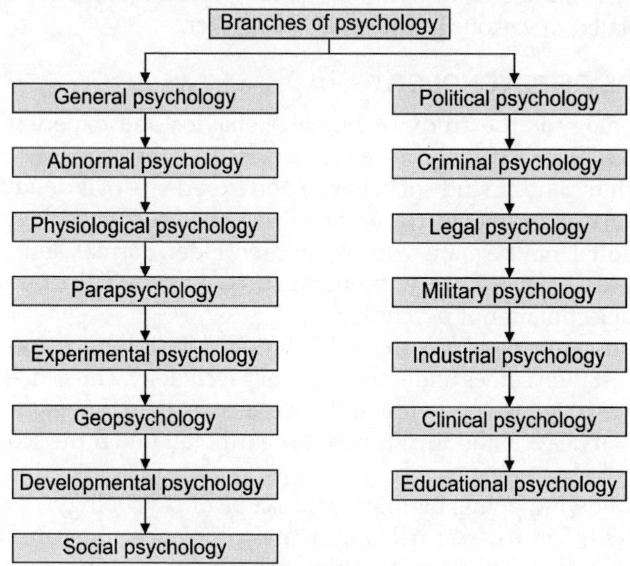

Fig. 1.2: Branches of psychology

- ***Geopsychology***: This branch deals with the relation of physical-environment especially weather, climate, soil and land space with behavior.

- ***Adult psychology***: This branch of psychology deals with various issues related to adults, i.e. growth and development, personality changes, attitude formation, interest, adjustment problem and their solution, etc. The knowledge of adult psychology helps in adult education, and understands the need of guidance and counseling for professionals to handle the adult problems.
- ***Correctional psychology***: This branch deals with the correction of many abnormal or correctional problems and activities and suggest relevant measures to correct them, i.e. undesirable and maladaptive behavior.
- ***Individual psychology***: Individual psychology deals with the study of individual differences among human being and their impact on outcome in achievement. Individual psychology studies the nature and cause of individual differences.
- ***Consumer psychology***: This branch is concerned with the various psychological aspects of consumer and related issues such as interest, attitude, bargaining and buying and selling related to various products in the market.

SCOPE OF PSYCHOLOGY

Psychology is the study of human behavior and experience of individual in relation to its environment. Whatever is concerned with the scientific study of behavior and experience of individual in relation to environment forms the subject matter of psychology. The individual may be man, woman, children, elder, normal, abnormal, social or unsocial, moral or immoral, social or antisocial, it becomes the subject matter of psychology.

Thus, we can say that the whole life of an individual in its every manifestation comes under the scope of psychology. Thus, the scope of psychology is very wide in the word of William James, 'all the chairs of heaven and furniture of the earth 'fall under the scope of psychology.

The following points highlights the scope of psychology:

- ***Mental processes***: All the mental processes like sensation, perception, attention, thinking, reasoning, learning, memory, imagination fall within the scope of psychology. As Prof Stout remarked, 'all the mental process which occurs in the life of a man fall in the scope of psychology'. We can observe various mental processes directly by looking inside our own mind.

- *Expression and behavior*: The appearance, expression and behavior of ourselves and other constitute subject matter of psychology. All the three forms of behavior or activities (i.e. cognitive, conative and affective behavior) are included in the scope of psychology.
- *Physiological process*: Various physiological process and bodily changes are studied in educational psychology. Various mental processes are accompanied by physiological changes and bodily activities. For example, emotions are accompanied by physiological changes in heart rate, pulse rate and blood pressure, digestive system, and hyper activity of glands and nervous system take place. Every emotional experience involves various physiological changes.

RELATION OF PSYCHOLOGY WITH OTHER SCIENCES

Psychology and Philosophy

At one time psychology was concerned with a part and parcel of philosophy. Just recently due to popularity of experimental methods, psychology has moved away from philosophy. Yet there is a close relationship between the two. Both psychology and philosophy attempt to interpret human behavior. Whatever truth philosophy discovers are in fact based on psychology. Even the most important branch of philosophy, i.e. epistemology is based on psychology. Epistemology investigates the origin of knowledge, its nature, validity and the way it is realized. This inquiry is never possible unless help is taken from psychological explanation. The metaphysical (metaphysics—a branch of philosophy) discussion are based on psychological interpretation of natural phenomena. Besides, epistemology and metaphysics, logic and ethics are important branch of philosophy.

Difference Between Psychology and Philosophy

- **Difference in nature:** Both psychology and philosophy differs from each other in nature. The nature of psychology is scientific and not philosophical as that of philosophy.
- **Difference in approach:** The main characteristic of philosophical approach is integral and synthetic. But as a science, psychology is analytical and limited in its stand point.
- **Difference in scope:** Behavior and experience of the individual is the scope of psychology. All aspects of knowledge are scope of philosophy.

- **Differences in method:** Scientific methods are used in psychology, i.e. experimental and observation method but the methods used in philosophy are concentration, meditation, logic and institution are subjective one.
- **Individual mind versus universal mind:** Psychology is concerned with individual mind while philosophy focuses on universal mind.

Psychology and Physiology

Relation between Psychology and Physiology

Physiology studies the function of the various organs like stomach, heart and systems, e.g. digestive or circulatory system of the body. Psychology studies the interaction of one system to another and their functions.

Psychology is the science of behavior and experience of the individual. Experiences of an individual are deeply connected with physiological process especially in various systems. Hence, psychology studies the physiological process in order to account for mental processes. Various organ of the body, system, muscular and glandular activities influence human behavior in one or another way. 'Healthy mind lives in a healthy body' is an ancient and well known proverb. Hence, psychology and physiology are closely related to each other.

Differences between Psychology and Physiology

- **Difference in scope:** The scope of psychology is mental activities and behavior whereas the physiology concerned to physical activities.
- **Difference in approach:** Psychology and physiology differ to each other in their approach. Psychology studies the reactions of the whole physical organism towards the other stimuli. Physiology studies the different physical activities separately.

Psychology and Sociology

Relation between Psychology and Sociology

Psychology intimately is related to sociology. Sociology is the science of society, i.e. of social relationship. It deals with the activities of a group of people taken as a whole. It studies social institution, customs traditions, culture, norms and other groups or behavior, etc. Psychology studies the human behavior which is influenced by customs traditions, culture, norms and social factors. Hence, there is considerable overlapping between the province of psychology and sociology.

- Both psychology and sociology are positive science
- Both are factual and use scientific methods for study
- In both, it is difficult to be absolutely objective
- Both have lesser power of prediction than other pure sciences.

Difference between Psychology and Sociology

- **Difference in attitude:** The attitude of psychologist is individualistic and that of sociologist is socialistic.
- **Difference in unit:** The unit of psychology is individual while sociology considers society or a group of people as a unit. Psychology studies man as individual, its interactions whereas sociology studies the society and its pattern and interaction as a whole.
- **Difference in methods:** Methods of psychology and sociology differ from each other.

Psychology and Education

Education and psychology are two distinct branches of knowledge; though they are closely related. Modern education is based on psychology. Child is imparted education after making a thorough study of his interest, aptitude, intelligence and personality. Without help of psychology various problems of education may not be solved. A preliminary knowledge of psychology has a great impact on various aspects of education.

Psychology is the science of behavior. Education is the modification of behavior. Education enables unfolding and developing the powers of the pupil and molding his character, personality and behavioral patterns. It is the process of helping him in making adjustment with social environment. As BN Jha said, 'education has to depend on psychological findings for what is done and how it is done.'

The knowledge of psychology is helpful in education in following ways:

- **Knowledge of innate nature:** Psychology helps in knowing the innate nature of the pupil. It helps to make the teaching successful while keeping in view the innate nature.
- **Knowledge of individual difference:** Psychology helps the teacher to understand the individual difference among pupil in

terms of interest, intelligence, achievements, motives and other traits. Knowledge of individual difference helps in handling the pupils and maintaining discipline.

- **Knowledge of learning:** Psychology helps in education, in understanding laws, methods, and factors of learning. Knowledge of related aspects of education enables a teacher in arousing attention and interest of the pupils. He can motivate the students for using effective methods of learning and memorization.
- **Psychology and aim of education:** Psychology helps the teacher in realization of the educational aims by helping him to bring about improvement in the quality of instruction by providing him insight into the child as interest, habits, emotions, intelligence and personality.
- **Psychology and time-table:** Time-table for imparting education can be prepared in accordance with sound psychological principles.
- **Psychology and discipline:** Psychology helps a teacher to maintain discipline in class by making judicious use of rewards and punishments.
- **Psychology and research:** Psychology has proved useful in the field of research. We can control, direct and predict the behavior of students on the basis of research studies in classroom teaching.

Psychology and Nursing

Nursing is the service to community. Knowledge of psychology helps health professional, i.e. nurses, doctors and other paramedical staff, to deal with patient and family members in a better way. As it is clear now that the behavior of an individual is subject matter of psychology. A sound knowledge of psychological theories and principles helps to understand the complex client behavior in clinical setting and enable to plan strategy to deal it effectively. There is a close relationship between nursing and psychology. Knowledge of psychology helps the students in various perspectives.

Relevance of Psychology to Nursing

Nurse is the central part of heath care team. A nurse perform varied types of duties and role in clinical setting to promote, restore and maintain health of their patient and significant others. A Nurse deals with different types of patients and their significant family members having different mental and physical problems. Thus, in performing the duties of nursing profession, it is very essential for a nurse to be more knowledgeable of different theories and principles of psychology to deal with the individual.

The knowledge of psychology helps the nurse in the following ways:

Box 1.1: Relevance of psychology to nursing

- Understand the patient
- Understand the relative and well wishers
- Get adjusted to professional environment
- Provide needed advise, guidance and support to the patient
- Provide quality care and nursing to patient
- Study during pre-service and/or in-service periods
- Maintain balance between personal and professionals life
- Help to conduct psychometric assessment
- Understand yourself

To help understand the relatives and significant of others: It is common problem for a nurse to deal the relatives and significant of others in the hospital. It becomes a challenging task to discipline them in agreeing to the hospital rules and having patience for expected outcomes of care. A sound knowledge of psychology may helps a nurse to deal with relatives and significant of others by understanding the reason of unusual behavior at hospital.

To help get adjusted to professional environment: It is very difficult for a novice nurse to adjust in hospital environment and with member of health care team. A nurse have to work in team and sometime all alone. The study of psychology will helps a nurse to understand the people around you and enable better adjustment with other health professional and in hospital.

To maintain balance between social and professional life: It is very essential for a nurse to maintain balance between social and professional life to provide quality care. The study of psychology helps to understand various aspects of personal, professional and social life and enables to adjust in different circumstances.

To help focus on study: Psychology helps a student nurse to focus on study by adhering with the principles, law and theories of perception, attitude, concentration, forgetting and motivation. Sound knowledge of above-mentioned psychological aspects helps a student nurse to achieve desired goals in professional life.

To help in conducting psychometric assessment: The study of psychology will help a nurse to learn and conduct the various psychometric assessment of the cognitive processes, emotional behavior, attention, personality traits, anxiety, stress and level of adjustment, etc.

To provide quality nursing care: An adequate knowledge and information of needs, desires, attitude, likes and dislikes of a patient helps a nurse to provide quality nursing care. The study of psychology may equip a nurse to have sufficient background knowledge of all attributes to take proper professional decision for providing needed nursing care to patient and his well wishers.

Community services: Knowledge and understanding of socio-cultural system of various social customs, traditions, taboos, and myths enable a community nurse to render effective community services and promote interpersonal affiliation and emotional integration between and within social group.

Promoting guidance and counseling: Knowledge of psychology helps in providing guidance and counseling services to person seeking solutions to their problems in the education, employment and personal life. A good person including nurse tries to understand all essential aspects of behavior and potentialities through various psychological measures and techniques and then suggest and tries possible ways and means to solve the difficulties of the person who has come for guidance and counseling services.

To understand development dynamics: By the knowledge of developmental psychology a nurse will be able to understand the various theories of growth and development milestones at various development stages.

Promoting mental health and hygiene: A nurse play vital role in promoting good mental health among his/her patients by the application of the knowledge of psychology. She will be able to understand different coping strategies to overcome stress, and various preventive measures to promote mental health and hygiene.

For better self-development: Psychology helps the individual to know his/her assets and limitation, abilities and shortcomings, habits and temperament, interest and attitude, etc. The understanding of self may lead one to set the level of his/her aspiration, change habits, seek self-control and strive for his/her adequate development and progress. It may help in proper catharsis and training of emotions, building up proper sentiments and decisions-making abilities and self-actualization in order to develop a balanced and integrated personality.

METHODS OF PSYCHOLOGY

Psychology, as we have pointed out before, is a science of behavior and experience of the individual in relation to environment, being a science, it has a special tools, procedures and or methods which helps in the collection of organization of facts or data. Methods save time, energy, efforts and efficiency. Some psychologists are in the view that because of these methods psychology is a science, and this very thing speaks of the importance of methods.

Meaning of method: The teaching method implies the system that we adopt in gaining knowledge of truth. Charles Gide said in this, 'in scientific language the term 'method' is used to designate the road that must be followed to lead the discovery of truth.'

According to Oxford Dictionary, 'method is a way of having something, system of procedure, orderliness and conscious of regularity etc'

Method and technique: Method is a wide-term than technique. In a method we may have many techniques. For example: free association and dream analysis are techniques of psychoanalytic method of Sigmund Freud.

List of Methods of Psychology

- Subjective observation/introspection
- Objective observation
- Experimental method
- Psychoanalytic method
- Clinical methods, i.e. case study method and developmental case study
- Correlation method
- Differential method (survey method)

Beside these methods, we have certain techniques and test like:

- Questionnaire
- Interview
- Rating scale
- Checklist
- Psychological test (intelligence test): Personality test, aptitude test, achievement test, anecdotal records, biographical record and auto-biographical records and sociometric techniques.

CHIEF METHODS OF PSYCHOLOGY

Introspection or Subjective Method

This is the oldest method of psychology. It could be the study method when psychology was defined as science of consciousness. It is derived from two words: 'intro' and 'spection'. 'Intro' means '*within*' and 'Spection' means '*looking*'. Hence, etymologically speaking introspection means '*looking within*'. Woodworth views that introspection is *self-observation*. Introspection is a developed form of self-consciousness. It can be defined as an inner observation of the mental events by the man himself at the time of occurrence.

Advantages of Introspection

Simplest and economic: It is one of the most simple and economic method and it does not require any laboratory, costly equipments or any other help because the individual will work as subject as well as object.

- **Private mental processes**: With the help of introspection, private mental processes which we do not want to share with other, can be explored and evaluated for their importance, i.e. sexual desires.
- **Time and place no bar:** It can be done at any place and at any time because individual mind is his/her own behavior.
- **Universal method:** In this method, we can study all types of individuals and their minds. The dacoits and smugglers cannot be studied by using experimental methods.
- **Improvement in personality:** It is useful method in bringing improvement in one's personality, for example, if there is any sort of abnormality, the individual can suggest some remedy to remove it by introspection.
- **Time honored method:** It is the time honored method which is available only in psychology not in other sciences.
- **Mind under intoxicants:** It is the best method for knowing the mind under intoxicants, feelings, emotions, sentiments, prejudice and pains.
- **Part of experimental report**: It forms an important part of experimental report. While writing experimental report we include introspective report of the subjects. Introspective report is essential.
- **Improvement in teaching:** The teacher can improve his/her teaching by suggesting the new method for teaching with the help of introspection.

Limitations of Introspection

- **Most subjective:** It is most subjective, personal and private method. The result cannot be objective and valid, and results cannot verify them. So it is unscientific method.
- **The observer and subject are same:** In this method mind is divided into two parts, i.e. knower and known. But practically mind cannot be divided into two parts, i.e. if we want to introspect anger, when we try to concentrate. In the other words of William James; 'it is trying to see the darkness by switching on light'. Introspection needs lot of constant practice and experience.
- **Not of universal application:** This method cannot apply on children, abnormal people, illiterate and animals.
- **Restricted to one person:** Introspection is limited to individual is own mental processes. We cannot have the view of other people. It is impossible to read the mind of others.
- **Subconscious and unconscious experience:** It is not applicable to unconscious and subconscious mind.
- **Birth and death experience:** Certain experience like birth and death cannot be introspected. Hence, it is inadequate to explore all human experiences.
- **Mental experiences:** Mental experiences are transitory and short lived. They evaporate as we begin to introspect them.
- No doubt, introspection has many limitations, but it is very easy and least expensive method of psychology. In experimental psychology, introspection report of the subject is recorded and experiment is regarded as incomplete without introspect report of the subject.

Objective Observation

This method of observation is old as introspection. It is also called naturalistic observation. Observation is of two types;

1. Controlled observation: Observation under controlled condition.
2. Uncontrolled observation: It is also called naturalistic observation.

Steps in the observation method

- *Observing the behavior*: The first step of observation start with perception or observation of behavior, e.g. observation of play school children.

- *Recording the observation*: The observed observation should be clearly and carefully recorded.
- *Analyzing the observation*: After the recording, the observation should be analyzed.
- *Interpreting and generalizing the observation*: This is the last step in observation process to give the meaning to data.

Characteristics of Good Observation

- Observation should be specific
- It should be systematic and planned
- It should be objective and scientific
- It should be whole.

Advantages of Observation Method

- **Objective and scientific:** This is more scientific and objective method of psychology than introspection.
- **Reliable and valid:** It is more valid and reliable method than introspection.
- **Simple and economic:** It is simple as well economic method as it does not need any laboratory and costly equipments.
- **Helpful for specific population:** Controlled observation is helpful to observe the behavior of children, abnormal person, animals, as individual or group.
- **Basis of experimental method:** It provides a ground basis for experimental method. Experimental method is nothing but objective observation under controlled or laboratory conditions.
- **Useful in educational situation:** With the help of this method of psychology, supervision of classroom teaching can be made; behavior of children can be detected, problem can be identified and outcome or corrective strategies can be planned.

Limitations of Observation Method

- **Trained observer:** It is very difficult to get a trained observer. Untrained observer may gather bias and irrelevant findings.
- **Subjective method:** Unplanned observation will be subjective in nature. It can be biased from observer side too. Sometimes observer may mix his/her likes and dislikes in observation.
- **Artificiality:** Sometimes, artificiality can come in the behavior. Presence of observer may change the behavior of subjects under observation.

- **Long wait:** Sometimes, observer has to wait for a very long time to occur the incident. For example, for observing the behavior of an angry child, an observer may have to wait for long time to happen angry behavior.
- **Difficulty in observing personal problems:** Some personal problems and experiences cannot be observed by observation, i.e. sexual experiences.
- **Difficulty in studying unconscious mind:** Observation is not helpful to record experience of unconscious mind.
- **Difficulty in studying internal behavior:** Observation only records the external behavior. It is not a good method to record internal behavior.

Though naturalistic observation has certain limitations yet it is considerable good method in the field of child psychology and educational psychology.

Experimental Method

Experimental method holds the central position in the psychology as well as in other sciences. It is experimentation which has the credit of bringing educational psychology to the level of exact sciences. Hence, modern psychology places the greatest emphasis as experimentation.

The experimental method first introduced by William Wundt in 1879 at Leipzig laboratory at Germany. In 1880, Ebbinghaus conducted many experiments on memory.

Essential for an Experiment

- **Psychological laboratory:** There should be fully equipped psychological laboratory with necessary equipments.
- **Experimenter:** There is an experimenter or experimenters.
- **Subject:** There is an individual subject or group of subject on whom the experiment is performed. In physical sciences experiments are performed on inorganic or dead subjects, whereas in psychology experiments are conducted on living organism.
- **Stimulus**: By stimulus we mean 'any physical force in the environment which impinges the organism to behave or to react'.
- **Response:** Response is the reaction to the stimulus. It can be defined as change in the behavior of organism which can be observed.

- **Variables:** The term 'variables' means which can be vary or change from one individual to another or one subject to another subject. Variables may be independent and dependent variables.
  - **Independent variable:** Independent variable is one which is systematically and independently manipulated by the experimenter to see the effect on dependent variable. It is also known as *input variable* or *treatment in medical research.*
  - **Dependent variable:** It is also known *outcome variable.* It is variable on which effect of independent variable is observed. For example, if we want to see the effect of green tea on blood pressure, here, green tea is independent variable and blood pressure is dependent variable.

Symbolically, it can be represented like this
Here,

X_1– Independent variable
O – Observation/intervention
X_2– Dependent variable

Steps followed in Psychological Experiments

A systematic experiment will follow following steps:

- **Defining the problem:** First of all problem should be defined clearly and experimenter should know what factors should be controlled and what to change.
- **Selection of subject:** That is, individual or group of subject on whom experiment has to perform.
- **Setting the material:** That is, selection of research instrument, place of experiment, etc.
- **Instructions to subject:** That is instructions to subject what to follow and what not to follow.
- **Procedure:** How the experiment will start and carried out, what steps to be followed, how much time it will take to complete.
- **Observing the response of subject:** Record the output of the subjects towards input variables.
- **Getting introspect report of the subject:** Self-evaluation of the report.
- **Collection of data and finding result:** Collect data by using appropriate research instrument and compile to make them meaningful.
- **Analysis and interpretation of data:** Analyze the data and interpret them to draw conclusion.
- Verifying the conclusions.

Advantages of Experimental Method

- **Reliable and valid:** Experimental method is most reliable, valid, systemic, most precise and most objective method of psychology.
- **Universal application:** This method is universally applicable to all, i.e. children, adult and even animals.
- **Wide application:** Experimental method is widely applicable in all branches of psychology especially in intelligence measurement, personality measurement, attitude measurement, individual difference and mental disorders.
- **Quantitative measurement:** It has introduced quantitative measurement in psychology. Individual studied internally by this method in quantitative manner like the study of emotion, motivation, learning and perception, etc.
- **Systematic and planned:** Experimental is systematically preplanned with full control on external environment to get accurate findings.
- **Verification:** Results of the experimental method can be verified.
- **Generalization:** Result of the experimental method can be generalized to other population.
- **Use in education:** Experimental method has wide implications in almost all areas of education, i.e. curriculum development, method of teaching, recruitment of teachers, guidance and counseling, etc.

Limitation of Experimental Method

- **Expensive:** It is very expensive and costly method among all methods of psychology. It needs lot of gadgets and equipments to handle experimental method.
- **Artificiality:** There is certain amount of artificiality of laboratory conditions and this artificiality hinder generalization of results.
- **Difficulty in controlling variables:** All variables cannot be controlled in experimental method. Lack of control on variables leads to spurious results.
- **Every phenomenon cannot be studied:** Certain phenomena cannot be studied under laboratory environment like cause of mortality and abnormal behavior, etc.

Although experimental method has certain limitations, yet it is very useful in almost all branches of educational psychology as well as in the various aspects of education.

Psychoanalytic Method

The psychoanalytic theory was postulated by Sigmund Freud (1856-1939). Freud (1939) who has been called as 'father of psychiatry' is credited as the first to identify the development by stages. He believed that an individual's basic charter is formed at an age of 5. Freud categorizes his theory according to following ways:
- Structure of personality, i.e. id, ego and superego
- Topography of mind, i.e. conscious, sub or pre-conscious and unconscious
- Psychosexual stages of development, i.e. oral, anal, phallic, latency and genital.

Structure of Personality

Freud organized the structure of personality into three main components; the id, ego and superego.
- **Id:** The id contain all our biological based drives—the way to eat, drink, eliminate, sex etc. The sexual energy that underlies these urges is called '*libido*'. The id operates according to the '*pleasure principle*'. That is, it desires to satisfy its urges immediately irrespective to rules, realities of life or moral of any kind. Id present at birth, it endows the infant with instinctual drives that seek to satisfy needs and achieve immediate gratification. Id drive behavior are impulses and may be irrational in nature.
- **Ego:** Ego begins to develop at an age, i.e. 4–5 month of birth. Ego works on 'reality principle'. The ego experiences the reality of the external world, understand it and work accordingly. A primary function of the ego is that mediator, which is to maintain harmony between the external world, the id and the super ego. Development of strong ego is a good sign of all round development of personality.
- **Superego:** This is also known as '*conscience*'. The super ego functions on 'ideal or perfection principle'. The super ego starts developing at age of 3 to 6 years. It internalizes the values and moral of family, friends and neighbors. Super ego helps to control the impulses of the id and delay the gratification impulses until the situation is appropriate. Improper development of super ego leads to low self-confidence in an individual.

According to Freud, all human behavior can be understood in terms of the dynamic equilibrium among id, ego and super ego.

The id demand to satisfy its immediate felt need irrespective of violation of norms of others and society, and ego will help to control the action of id by delaying or compromising the situation. A well balanced personality is governed by the ego and psychopathic by id. The aim of psychoanalysis is to restore the balance, where id was 'there shall be ego'.

Topography of Mind

Freud said that human brain is a storehouse of information and on the basis of recall of information; brain is combination of the following three parts:

1. **The conscious:** The conscious mind is concerned to the information which can be freely recalled and for recalling of these information effort are not needed. It covers only 10% of total brain.
2. **The unconscious:** This is the largest portion of the brain. Freud claimed that the mind is like an ice-berg in that most of its portion is hidden beneath the surface and called unconscious mind. It covers around 80% of total human brain. It stores all the information related to repressed conflicts like desires, wishes, motives, feelings and drives–many of which may be related to sex and aggression, etc. This hidden treasure is responsible for most of the human behavior.
3. **Sub or pre-conscious:** This section of brain contain only around 10% of total brain. Some of the daily information may goes and store in the subconscious mind. Recalling the information from unconscious mind need some effort and time. Then, it is often referred as '*tip on tongue*'.

Psychosexual Stage of Personality Development

Freud believed that initial stage of perssonality development is an important predictor of adult personality. He described five stages of personality development also known as psychosexual stage of personality development. He places emphasis on first five year of life and believed characteristics development during these five years had great impact on adult personality. Fixation on early stage of development will almost certainly result in psychopathology.

- **The oral stage (0–18 months):** In this stage, mouth represents the first sex organ for providing pleasure to the child. Focus of energy is mouth. During this stage behavior is directed by id. At the age of 4–6 month, the development of ego begins and child starts to view the self as separate from the mothering figure.

- **The anal stage (18 months–3 years):** The interest of the child shift from mouth to the excretory organ, i.e. anal or urethra. During this stage id is slowly brought under the control of ego. The child enjoys this stage by passing or holding the body waste material through anus or urethra. The anal stage end with the toilet training.
- **The phallic stage (3–6 years):** The major task during this stage is the identification with parents of the same sex and development of sexual identity. The child drives pleasure by stimulating genitalia. The development of oedipus complex (male) and electra complex (female) take places during this stage. Freud described it as an unconscious desire to eliminate the parent of same sex and to possess the parent of the opposite sex.
- **The latency stage (6–12 years)**: At this stage, children show a distinct preference for same sex relationship, even rejecting of opposite sex.
- **The genital stage (13–30 years)**: At this stage, heterogeneous sexual attraction begin, libido is reawakened as genital organ mature. Individual focus is on relationship with member of the opposite sex. Sexual maturity develops and gender identity also completely developed.

Clinical Methods

It is one of the most important methods of psychology to collect the detailed information on the problem of the maladjustment and deviant cases. This technique borrowed from medical sciences in the field of social sciences. The main objective of this method is to study individual case or cases of groups to detect and diagnose their specific problem in order to suggest therapeutic measure to rehabilitate them in their own environment. To collect data pertaining to case, it utilizes various techniques to compile relevant information which has some direct and indirect links with the problem of case. The case is studied intensively in temporal sequence from birth of the individual to the present manifestation of the problems in overt activities.

The objective of the clinician is to detect or to go into unconscious of the individual to pinpointing local underlying cases of the problem and to suggest remedial measures. The complete and detailed study of a case may involve the use of observation, interview, medical examination and use of various psychological test, i.e. intelligence, personality, aptitude, interest etc. The clinician collects the information about the case in totality. Common used clinical methods are:

***The clinical case study*:** This method is specifically important in various emotional problems, various disabling conditions like physical, speech, learning difficulties, mental illness, delinquency and other behavior problems.

Case study method generally used in case of a person suffering from mental disorder or behavioral disorders. It is used to collect the different types of information of the individual to identify the condition influencing his behavior. In other words, in case study method, the past and present situation of the individual is explored to find out the factors influencing his behavior. In this method an attempts is made to explore the cause of present motives or intention of an individual. Hence, it is systematic, complete and intensive history of the individual, his family background, his physical, social, emotional, intellectual and personal development. Nothing is left which is likely having effect on present conditions of the case to develop an in-depth understanding of the case.

So, the preparation of case study is not a work of single individual whereas it is a combine adventure of professionals and personals. Some important steps of this method are given here:

- **Preliminary information:** name, age, gender, education, social status, family background, family type and size, number of children etc.
- **Past history:** From conception of at least from infancy to till today. Main emphasis is on developmental milestones and achievements of the person.
- **Present history/condition:** This may be collected under following headings; physical, mental, social, emotional, interest. School achievement, job achievement, etc.

These are the tentative list of various sources from which information may be collected to prepare a case history/study. In brief, we can say that case study method helps to understand the root cause of problem and it is very valuable method in suggesting remedial measures to rehabilitate them.

Developmental case study: Developmental case study or genetic method generally used to collect data in the following time frame pattern to understand development structure of the individual.
Longitudinal approach: In this approach information are collected over a period of long time to understand the various changes in the case at different period of interval i.e. from birth to adolescent stage.
Cross-sectional approach: In which we select sample from different age level to study the specific aspects of development.

Steps Involved in Case Study

A psychologist follows following steps in case study method:
- **Selection of case:** That is, a case with any psychological and behavioral problems.
- **Collection of information:** Information are collected from multiple sources like patient, significant family members, teachers, friends, and records, etc.
- **Analysis of data:** Once information are collected, it is compiled to analyze and make them meaningful.
- **Removing the causes:** That is, application of remedial or adjustment measures.
- **Follow-up the cases:** That is a short or long term follow-up is designed to determine the effectiveness of remedial or adjustment measures applied.

Characteristics of a Good Case Study

A comprehensive case study should have following characteristics:
- **Completeness:** A case study must be complete and comprehensive in all aspects. It should cover all the necessary details needed to rule out diagnosis.
- **Continuity of data:** The information collected must be in the sequence like background information, present chief complaints, present history of illness and so on.
- **Valid information:** The information collected must be valid. Collected information should be cross checked with the information of informant or case sheet of the patient.
- **Confidential recording:** A case study should keep all the information of an individual private and confidential.

Scientific synthesis and analysis: Once the case study is over, the recorded information should be synthesized and analyzed to rule out the diagnosis.

Uses of Case Study Method

- **Comprehensive study:** Case study method useful for comprehensive and complete analysis of an individual
- **Helpful in diagnosis:** This method is helpful for findings causes of maladjustment of a person and then findings out suitable treatment.
- **Identify school problems:** This method is useful in the study of school problems such as severe reading disability, sever stemmer, stuttering, chronic delinquent and severe emotional disturbances, etc.

Limitations of Case Study

- **Subjective method:** It is a subjective method. A person who collects information may project his own problems, plans, ideas, attitudes, values into the report.
- **Lengthy method:** It is lengthy method and time-consuming method of psychology.
- **Need trained experts:** A comprehensive case study is the result of effort of a trained person.
- **Difficult to prepare and interpret:** Sometimes, it is very difficult to prepare case study as patient family members will not cooperate. It also takes lot of time and help of experts to interpret the results.
- **Limited scope:** The case study method has limited scope of generalization. This method is not of universal application.
- **Depends on memory:** Largely the methode of case study method depends on memory. Sometimes, recalling the recorded information may be inaccurate or over inter operated. Memory may fail or deceive the person.

Correlation Method

This is non-experimental research method. A correlation is defined as a relationship between two variables such that when change in one variable leads to change in another variable. For example, there is a strong relationship between the use of drugs in first trimester and development of mental retardation in fetus. The more the use of drug leads to more cognitive disturbance in a child.

Differential Method (Survey Method)

It is used to study individual difference among individuals. Studies in the field of psychology make an extensive use of statistical survey which is based of sampling by collecting data through direct observation. This method makes use of various techniques of collecting data, i.e. test, questionnaire, observation, interview and use of statistic in analyzing the data in order to reach on conclusions. Survey methods are broadly classified in the following three categories which share common features of carrying out their observation on lager size samples belong to defined population.

- **The filed study:** A field experiment may be defined as scientific investigation carried out in the field which involves direct manipulation of some independent variables. The field study is conducted in natural settings, i.e. classroom teaching learning and curriculum development.
- **Developmental survey:** Although developmental survey and developmental clinical study looks similar in method but differ in purpose. Clinical developmental method is concerned to an individual but developmental survey cover a large population to study the typical pattern of change in growth and development of behavior over a specific period of time span. Like developmental clinical methods, development survey may be longitudinal or cross sectional in nature. For example, we can say about the development of intelligence in culturally disadvantage of children from birth to 5 years using either longitudinal or cross sectional method.
- **Differential survey:** O'Neil refers two examples of differential survey which he said as those concerned with establishing typical difference between individual, and between classes of individual. The study conducted by Klinberg into difference in individual between racial and national groups in Europe come under differential survey.

Limitations of Survey Method

Survey method limitations lies under the followings:

- **Sample error**: Sometime sample are not true representative of the population. In case of biased sample result of the survey study is limited to that population and hinders the generalization over other population.
- **Lack of cooperation:** This is most significant source of error in differential survey. Sometime, researcher is not able to get honest cooperation of the subject in survey and this leads to false results.

- **Inadequate sample size:** This is particularly true for survey. An ideal survey needs large sample size to generalize the result over other population. For example, sample size for mental ability test and personality test.

Suggested Reading

- Anthikad J. Psychology for Graduate Nurses, 4th edn. New Delhi, Jaypee Brothers Medical Publishers (P) Ltd, 2008.
- Bhatia BD, Craig M. Elements of Psychology and Mental Health, 1st edn. Hyderabad, Orient Longman, 2006.
- Morgan CT, King RA, Weiz JR, et al. Introduction to Psychology, 7th edn. New Delhi. Tata McGraw Hill Publishing Company Ltd, 2007.
- Plotnik R. Introduction to Psychology, 5th edn. USA, Wadsworth Publishing Company, 1999.
- Sreevani R. Textbook of Psychology. Jaypee Brothers Medical Publishers (P) Ltd, 2008.

REVIEW QUESTIONS

SHORT-ESSAY TYPE QUESTIONS

1. Define psychology. Enlist the branches of psychology.
2. Enlist various methods used in psychology. Discuss experimental method in detail.
3. Discuss the importance of psychology in nursing.
4. Explain the scope of psychology.
5. Explain survey method in detail.

MULTIPLE CHOICE QUESTIONS

1. Who established the psychology lab in German University?
   a. Sigmund Freud b. BF Skinner
   c. Louis Pasture d. Wilhelm Wundt
2. Who is father of psychology?
   a. Ivan Pavlov b. Wilhelm Wundt
   c. JB Watson d. Kort Koffa

3. 'The study of the mind should focus on how it allows us to adapt to surrounding'. This statement is proposed by which psychologist?
   a. Kort Koffa
   b. Wilhelm Wundt
   c. BF Skinner
   d. William James
4. Which of the following perspective is known as third space of psychology?
   a. Psychoanalysis
   b. Behaviorism
   c. Cognitive psychology
   d. Humanism
5. First psychology laboratory established at:
   a. Leipzig, Germany
   b. Toronto, Canada
   c. Columbia, USA
   d. Italy
6. Superego is also known as:
   a. Self
   b. Ideal self
   c. Perfection
   d. Conscience
7. Which of the following is the most oldest method of psychology?
   a. Experimental method
   b. Survey method
   c. Introspection/subjective method
   d. Observational method
8. Who introduced the method of introspection?
   a. Watson
   b. Pavlov
   c. BF Skinner
   d. Wilhelm Wundt
9. Which of the following method will be used to find the relationship of one variable to another?
   a. Experimental method
   b. Survey method
   c. Case study
   d. Introspection
10. The literal meaning of word 'psychology' is:
    a. Study of behavior
    b. Study of mind
    c. Study of soul
    d. Study of appearance
11. Who developed Individual psychology?
    a. Freud
    b. Spearman
    c. GW Allport
    d. Alfred Adler
12. Psychology's major contribution in education lie in:
    a. Providing a scientific foundation for the art of teaching.
    b. Defining the goals on which the teacher should strive.

c. Identifying potentially successful educational procedures.
d. Comparing the relative effectiveness of various teaching procedures.

13. The behaviorists believed:
    a. Psychology should emphasize the study of healthy people.
    b. Psychology should only study observable and objectively described acts.
    c. Psychology should study the self examination of inner ideas and experiences.
    d. All of the above

ANSWER KEY

1.	d	2.	b	3.	b	4.	d	5.	a	6.	d	7.	c
8.	d	9.	a	10.	c	11.	d	12.	d	13.	b		

Biology of Human Behavior

Chapter 2

INTRODUCTION

The definition of psychology depict as a science of human behavior which is related to behavior and the mind. Physiological psychology is the branch of psychology which studies the effect of human physiology on human behavior. In order to study the human behavior, it is necessary to have a general understanding of the nervous system. Nervous system is not fully developed at birth, it rather grows and change in structure and function gradually. The simultaneous function of different parts and unit of the nervous system help us to behave like human. The structure and function of nervous system is so complex and no other species and machine can substitute it.

NERVOUS SYSTEM

The nervous system is the machine by which our behavior is controlled and regulated. Here a brief description of different part of nervous system is given.

Neuron

Neuron are the basic building blocks of the nervous system. The whole nervous system is made up of neuron along with supporting tissues and blood vessels. The functions of neurons also vary. The neuron are of different types; afferent (sensory) neuron, efferent (motor), and inter neuron or association neuron. These neurons are of various sizes, shapes and filled with different types of chemical called neurotransmitter. Neurons are interconnected to other each other and able to transmit the information from one neuron to another neuron. Like other cell in human body nerve cells also engaged in energy production for its existence.

Parts of Neuron

Neuron has the following parts:

- Axon
- Dendrites
- Cell body or stoma
- Terminal buttons (knob)

The control center of the neuron is located in its stoma or cell body. It has a single, centrally located nucleus with large nucleolus. The cytoplasm contains mitochondria, lysosomes, a golgi complex, numerous inclusions and an extensive rough endoplasmic reticulum and cytoskeleton. Cytoskeleton consist of a dense mesh of microtubules and neurofibrils (bundle of action filaments) that compartmentalize the rough endoplasmic reticulum into dark staining regions called Nissl bodies, unique to neuron. Some of neuron usually give rise to a few thick processes that branch into a vast number of dendrites. The dendrites are the primary site of receiving signals from other neurons. Some neurons only have one dendrites and some other have thousands. Dendrites are the receiving or input portion of a neuron. The plasma membranes of dendrites contain numerous receptors sites for binding chemical messages from other cells. Dendrites are usually short, tapering and highly branched.

The single axon of a neuron propagates nerve impulses through neurotransmitters via synapses to other neurons. Axon after joint to the cell body at a cone shaped elevation called the axon-hillock.

Classification of Neurons

Both structural and functional classification used to classify the various neurons in the body.

- **Structural classification:** This classification based on number of processes extending from the cell body.
  - **Multipolar neuron:** These neurons usually have several dendrites and one axon. Most neurons of human body are of this kind.
  - **Bipolar neuron:** This kind of neurons have one main dendrites and one axon. They are found in eye, ear and olfactory part of brain.
  - **Unipolar neuron:** In this kind of neuron, dendrites and axon fused together to form a continuous process that emerges

from the cell body. Neurons of sensory organ like skin for touch, temperature, pressure and pain are unipolar kind of neurons.

- **Functional classification:** These neurons are classified on the basis of directions of conveying of nerve impulses.
- **Sensory (afferent) neuron:** These types of neuron convey the sensory impulses from organ to spinal cord to central nervous system.
- **Motor (efferent) neuron:** These neurons conveyed the nerve impulses from central nervous system to spinal cord to final destination or organ.
- **Inter neuron or association neuron:** These neurons located between sensory and motor neurons. These neurons process incoming sensory impulses and then elicit motor response by achieving the appropriate motor neurons.

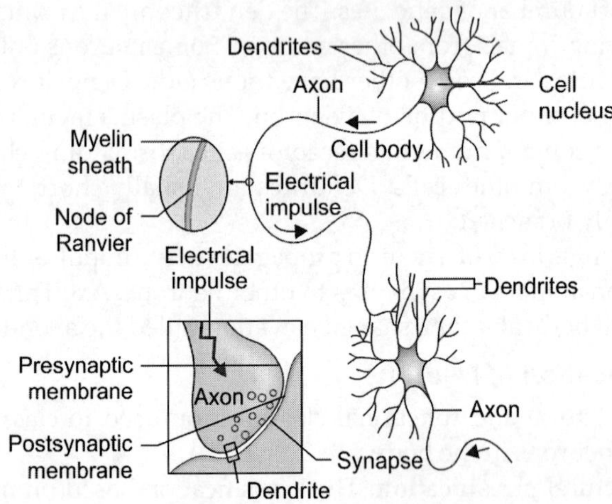

Fig. 2.1: Structure of neuron

Nerve Impulse Conduction

Like muscle fibers, neurons are electrically excitable. They communicate one another by using two types of electrical signals.

1. **Graded potentials:** Graded potential are used for short distance communication.
2. **Action potentials:** Action potential used for long distance communication.

Process of Nerve Impulse Transmission

To understand the function of graded and action potentials, consider the following steps:

- As you touch the object, a graded potential develop in a sensory receptors in the skin of the fingers.
- The graded potential action stimulate the axon of the sensory neurons to form a nerve action potentials, which travel along the axon into the central nervous system and ultimately causes the release of neurotransmitter at synopsis within interneuron.
- The neurotransmitter stimulate the interneuron to form a graded potential in its dendrites and cell body.
- In response to the graded potential, the axon of the interneuron form nerve action potential. The nerve action potential travel along the axon with the release of neurotransmitters at synaptic level.
- Once the stimuli reach to cerebral cortex, the outer part of the brain are activated, perception occurs and you are able to feel the object with the fingers.

The production of graded potential and action potentials depends on two basic features of plasma membrane of excitable cells; the existence of resting membrane potentials and the presence of specific types of ion channels like most other cell in the body, the plasma membrane of excitable cells exhibits a membrane potential, an electrical potential difference across the membrane. In excitable cell, this voltage is termed as resting membrane potential. The membrane potentials is like voltage stored in a battery. If you connect positive and negative terminals of a battery, the electron flow will start.

An action potentials or impulse is segments of a rapidly occurring event that decrease and reverse the membrane potential and then eventually restore it to the resting state. An action potential has two main phases: depolarizing phase and repolarizing phase. During the depolarizing phase, the negative membrane potential become more negative and reaches zero, and then become positive. During the repolarizing phase, the resting potential reaches to its usual stage—70 mv. Two types of voltage gated channels open and then close during an action potential of the first channel then open, the voltage gated Na^+ channels, allow Na^+ to rush into cell, which cause the repolarizing phase. Then voltage gated K^+ channels open, allowing K^+ to flow out, resulting the repolarizing phase. The generation of an action potential depends on whether a particular stimulus is able to bring the membrane potentials to threshold.

Refractory period: The period of time after an action potential begin during which an excitable cell cannot generate another action potential in response to normal threshold stimulus is called the refractory period. During the absolute refractory period, even a very strong stimulus cannot initiate a second action potential.

Neurotransmitters

Neurotransmitters are particularly important message carrier between two synaptic links. Deficiency and excess of a neurotransmitter can produce related behavioral changes. Some important neurotransmitters are listed in Table 2.1.

Table 2.1: Neurotransmitters and their functions

Serotonin	Maintain sleep, eating, mood state and pain
Gamma-aminobutyric acid (GABA)	Moderate eating, aggression, sleeping and memory process
Acetylcholine	Regulate muscle movements and cognitive functions
Dopamine	Regulate movements and coordination, emotions and other activities
Endorphins	Regulate pain and pleasant, mood elevating activities.

COMPONENTS OF NERVOUS SYSTEM

The nervous system is one of the smallest and the most complex of all 11 body system. The intricate network of billions of neurons and even more neuroglias is organized into two main sub-divisions.

1. **The Central Nervous System (CNS):** The central nervous system (CNS) consists of brain and spinal cord. The brain is the part of CNS that is located in the skull and contains about 11 billion neurons. The spinal cord connected to brain through foramen magnum of the occipital bone and is encircled by the bone of the vertebral columns. Spinal cord contains about 100 million of neurons.
2. **The Peripheral Nervous System (PNS):** The Peripheral nervous system (PNS) consists of all nervous tissues outside of the CNS. Components of PNS include nerve cells (31 pair spinal nerves and 12 pair cranial nerves), ganglia, metric plexus and sensory receptors. The PNS is again divided in somatic (autonomic) nervous system and enteric nervous system.

The Brain: Brain is one of the most complex and magnificent organ in the human body. Brain gives us awareness about surrounding environment. It controls our muscle movements, the secretion of our glands and even our breathing, body temperature and all other bodily functions. Every creative thought, feeling, and pain is controlled by mind. Brain is the store house of our daily learning. The brain is composed of the following three parts:

1. **The Cerebrum:** This is the largest part of brain and composed of left and right hemisphere. It perform high functions like interpreting touch, vision, hearing, as well as speech, language, emotion, learning and control of movements.
2. **The Cerebellum:** This is located under the cerebrum. This involves in muscle coordination, maintenance of posture and balance.
3. **The Brainstem:** Brainstem consist of three parts—Midbrain, Pons and Medulla oblongata. It acts as rely center connecting the cerebellum and cerebrum to the spinal cord. It perform many autonomic factors such as breathing, heart rate, body temperature, wake and sleep cycles, digestion, sneezing, coughing, vomiting and swallowing. Ten of twelve cranial nerves originate in the brainstem.

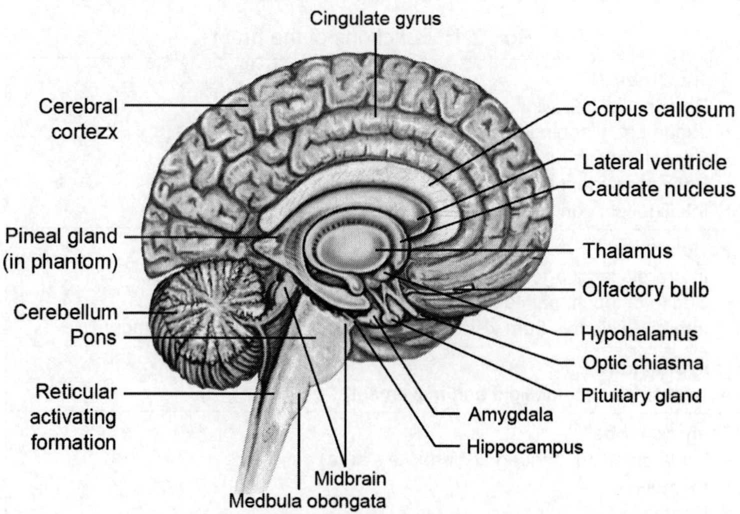

Fig. 2.2: Brain anatomy

The surface of the brain has folded appearance called the cortex. The cortex contains about 70% of the 100 billion nerve cells. The nerve cells bodies color the cortex gray-brown giving it its name grey matter. Beneath the cortex, a long connecting fiber between neurons, called axons, is located, which make up the white matter. The folding of the cortex increases the brain surface area allowing more neurons to fit inside the skull and enabling higher functions. Each fold is called a gyrus and each grove between fold is called sulcus. These are the names for the folds and grooves that help define brain regions.

Hemispheres of the Brain

The right and left hemispheres of the brain are joined a bundle of fibers called the corpus callosum that delivers massage from one side to other side. Each hemisphere controls the opposite side of the body. For example, if a brain tumor is located on the right side of the brain, your left arm or leg may be weak or paralyzed. No functions of the hemispheres are shared in general. The left hemisphere controls speech, comprehension, arithmetic, and writing. The right hemispheres control creativity, spatial activity, artistic and numerical skills. The left hemisphere is dominant in hand use and language about 92% people.

Box 2.1: Functions of the brain

Frontal lobe
- Personality, behavior and emotions
- Judgment, planning and problem-solving
- Speech, speaking, writing (Broca's area)
- Body movement (motor strip)
- Intelligence, concentration, self-awareness

Parietal lobe
- Interprets language, words
- Sense of touch, pain and temperature
- Interprets signals from vision, hearing, motor, sensory and memory

Occipital lobe

Interpret vision (color, light and movement)

Temporal lobe
- Understanding language (Wernicke's area)
- Memory
- Hearing
- Sequencing and organization

Lobes of the Brain

The cerebral hemispheres have distinct fissures, which divide the brain into lobes. Each hemisphere has 4 lobes—frontal, temporal, parietal and occipital. Each lobe may be divided, once again; into areas that serves as various specific functions. It is important to understand that each lobe of the brain does not function alone. There is very complex relationship between the lobes of the brain and between the right and left hemisphere.

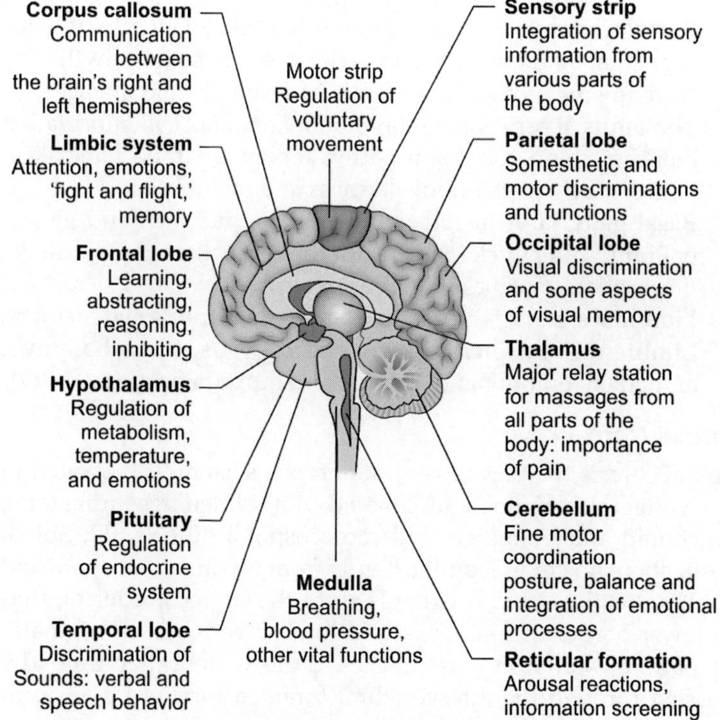

Fig. 2.3: Structure of brain

Messages with the brain are arrived along the pathway and can travel from one gyrus to another, from one side of the brain to another, and to structure found deep in the brain (i.e. thalamus and hypothalamus).

Deep Brain Structures

- **Hypothalamus:** Hypothalamus is located in the floor of third ventricle and is the master control of the autonomous system.

It plays an important role in controlling behavior like hunger, thirst, sleep, sexual desire. It also regulates body temperature, blood pressure, emotions and secretions of hormones.

- **Pituitary gland:** It lies in a small pocket of bone at the sella turcica. The pituitary gland is connected to the hypothalamus of the brain by the pituitary stalk. It is also known as master gland as it regulate other glands of human body. It secretes hormones that controls sexual development, promote bone and muscle growth, response to stress and fight disease.
- **Pineal gland:** It is located behind the third ventricle. It helps to regulate the body's internal clock and circadian rhythm by secreting melatonin. It has a role in sexual development.
- **Thalamus:** It serves as a relay station for almost all information that comes and goes to the cortex. It plays an important role in pain sensation, attention, alertness and memory.
- **Basal ganglia:** It includes the caudate, putamen and globus pallidus. Tube nuclei work with the cerebellum to coordinate fine motions, such as finger tip movement.
- **Limbic system:** It is center of or emotions, learning and memory. Limbic system includes cingulate gyrus, hypothalamus, amygdala (emotional reactions) and hippocampus (memory).

Spinal Cord

Spinal cord is the part of central nervous system. It is located in the vertebral columns and covered by the meninges (diameter, arachnoid and piamater) and cerebrospinal fluid (CSF). Spinal cord, about 45 cm in length extends from medulla oblongata and continues till coccyx. It extends from the upper border of atlas to lower border of first or second lumbar vertebra. It originates 31 pairs of spinal nerves that leave the vertebral columns by passing through the intervertebral foramen formed by adjacent vertebra.

Autonomous Nervous System (ANS)

Autonomous or involuntary part of the nervous system controls the autonomic functions (i.e. blood pressure, rate of breathing) of the body. This system works automatically without a person is conscious effort. Although stimulation may not occur voluntarily, the individual may be conscious of its effects. The two divisions have structural and functional differences. They usually work in an opposite manner, thereby maintaining functions. For example, the sympathetic division increases blood pressure, and parasympathetic division decreases it. The autonomous nervous system has two main divisions:

Divisions of Nervous System

Sympathetic nervous system: Sympathetic activity tends to predominate in stressful or emergency situation—flight or fight response. Thus, it increases heart rate and force of contractions, and widen the airway to make breathing easier. The sympathetic system is connected to the spinal cord and carries massages to the muscle and glands.

Parasympathetic nervous system: Parasympathetic activity during ordinary or rest stage. It slows heart rate and decreases blood pressure. It stimulates the digestive tract to processes of food and eliminates wastes.

Two chemical messengers (neurotransmitter), acetylcholine and nor epinephrine, are used to communicate within the autonomic nervous system. Acetylcholine has parasympathetic effect and nor epinephrine has sympathetic effect.

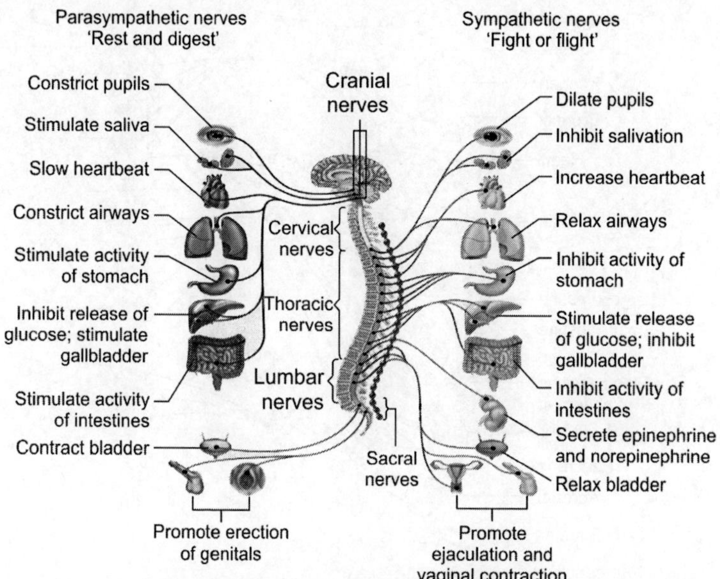

Fig. 2.4: Sympathetic and parasympathetic system

Table 2.2: Sympathetic and parasympathetic system

Division	Effects
Sympathetic	• Increase heart rate and force of contractions • Increase release of energy stored in the livers • Speed at which energy is used to perform body functions while a person is at rest (basic metabolic rate) • Increase muscle strength • Widen the airway to make the breathing easier • Cause sweaty palms • Decrease functions that are less important in an emergency (such as digestion and urination) • Control the release of semen (ejaculation)
Parasympathetic	• Stimulate the digestive tract to processes food and eliminate wastes (in bowel movement) • Slow the heart rate • Reduce blood pressure • Control erections

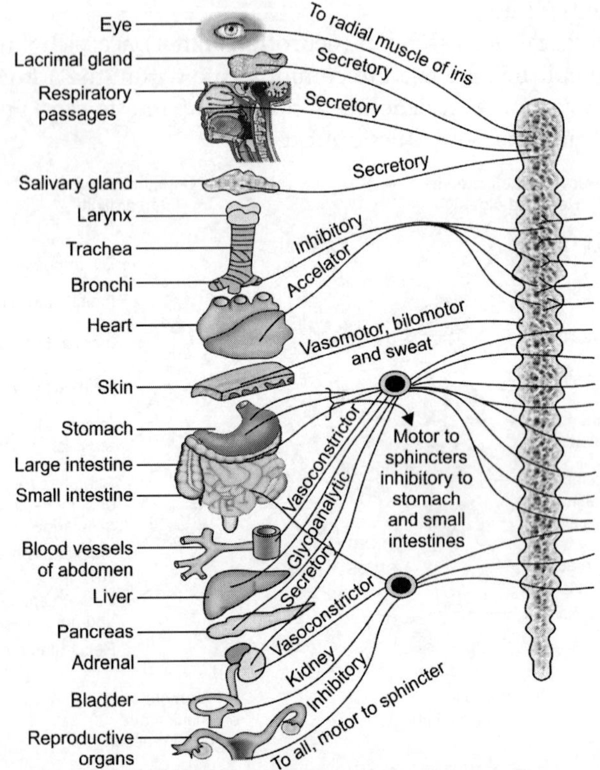

Fig. 2.5: Structure of spinal cord

BODY–MIND RELATIONSHIP

Brain and Behavior

Psychology defined as a scientific study of human behavior. The study of human behavior has a strong physiological and anatomical relation with brain. The entire human behaviors is effectively managed and controlled by human mind. All physiological and psychological influences are result of judgment of brain. For understanding the ultimate relationship between body and mind, it is mandatory to understand that:

- Body and mind are inseparable
- Body and mind depends on each others
- Body and mind interactions are responsible for change in behavior under certain disease conditions.

Body and mind inseparable: Previously, it was considered that mind and body both are separate as mind represents mental activity and body represent physical activity. However, how it is well accepted that both are inseparable. Mind is not reality, it is hypothetical construction and give rise to many acts and activities, commonly named as mental activities. It is not possible to imagine the existence of mind without body.

Body and mind act on each others: Mind and body affect each others. It is evidenced that the presence of any disturbances in bodily functions leads to disturbances in mind or mental functions in one or another way. For example, excessive tired and fatigue decreases attention and concentration on the task. Malfunctioning of various body systems may interfere with mental functioning, i.e. constipation may cause irritability.

Modulation Process in Health and Illness

Body is represented by various physical status and body functions. Our nervous system and various glands play an important role in thinking, feelings and doing. All human behavior is the result of coordination of brain and other body systems. Changes in one bodily systems will affect the other part in one and another way. Modulation refers to the process of regulating or varying the state of health and illness of an individual.

Effects of Physical Condition on Mental Functioning

- Increase blood pressure may cause mental excitement
- Severe pain and fatigue may reduces the concentration level

- Chronic illness may cause depression
- Malfunctioning of the endocrine glands may exert influence on other system, i.e. hypothyroidism leads to low mental status.

Effects of Mental Stress

- Condition on physical functioning
- Long-term unpleasant emotional state may cause irritability or headache
- Chronic stress may responsible for gastric ulcer and ulcerative colitis and other physical illness
- Repressed thoughts and feelings can cause heart attack or other physical conditions like migraine headache.

So, we can say that a nurse should understand the importance of body mind relationship. She should also understand the influence of change in mental system on physical functioning and vice-versa. It is mandatory for a nurse to know the physical and mental status of a patient to provide holistic care.

GENETIC AND BEHAVIOR

Genetics is the science of coming into being. Genetics is the branch of biological sciences which deals with the transmission of characteristics from parents to offspring. Genetics also defined as the sciences which deal with the study of hereditary and variations. The study of influence of an organism's genetics composition on its behavior is called behavior genetics or psychogenetic. George Mendel is known as father of genetics. His well known and popular experiment on the pea plants is an enormous invention in the history of genetics. Hereditary play an important role in behavior development modulation and expression. Almost all behavior affected by our genetic make-up. Quite often genes may predispose a person to develop peculiar traits but full expressions of the characteristics depend on environmental factors. Given the same environment for two different human beings may lead to changes in physical morphology. For example, a person who inherits 'tall' genes will be tall and a person who inherits 'short' genes will be short. But, if the first person malnourished during nurture and the second person is well nourished, they may be of same height. Because an individual's genotype does not always correspond obliviously or directly to what is expressed, the term phenotype is used when referring to the outwards expressions of traits. For example, people with an inherited tendency to gain weight (genotype) may or may not become obese (phenotype) depending on their diet, exercise and overall health.

The goal of behavior genetics is to identify the ways in which genes contributed to intelligence, temperament, talent, motivations, emotions, personality and predispose towards psychological and neurological disorders in future. Of course, genes do not directly cause behavior, rather, they affect the development and operation of nervos system and endocrine system, which, in turn influence behavior and mental processes.

Human Behavior Genetics

For oblivious reason, scientists cannot conduct strain or selection studies with human being. But there are many other ways to study genetic issue indirectly. To obtain a clear picture of the influence of hereditary and environment, psychologist often use twin studies, identical twins, develop from a simple fertilized ovum and are, therefore identical in genetic make-up at conception. For example, in schizophrenia, the twin studies indicate that success of developing schizophrenia to other twin will be almost 50%, for fraternal twin, the chances are about 15%.

Mechanism of Hereditary

The human life begins with the conception of ovum and sperm and start with a single cell called zygote. Both sperm and ovum has their own distinct gene pattern. An ovum consist 23 pairs of chromosome given by father and mother equally. A female have 23 pairs of XX chromosome and father have 22 pairs of XX chromosomes plus two single chromosome represented by X and Y and XY are called sex chromosomes. The 46 chromosomes in every cell containing 20,000 to 25,000 genes, creates a unique genetic 'blue print' or 'genotype'.

Genes are composed of deoxyribonucleic acids (DNA), as complex organic molecules that looks like chain twisted around each other in a double helix pattern. Like chromosomes, genes also occur in pairs, with one being dominant and one being recessive.

For example, in case of eye color, brown eye are dominants; all other colors (blue, green and hazel) are recessive.

Hereditary is the basis for development of human personality. Any molding and changes in the gene pattern will influence the personality. Many aspects of human behavior and personality like height, weight, color of eye, intelligence level, and social behavior are determined by genetic pattern. Hereditary is the only source of similarities and difference among individuals.

GLANDULAR CONTROL OF BEHAVIOR

Human body has a number of glands which plays an important role in regulating various bodily activities (i.e. digestion, metabolism, temperature, elimination etc). Broadly, these glands are classified under following headings:

- Ductless or endocrine glands
- Duct glands

The ductless or endocrine glands release a chemical substance in blood called hormones. These hormones carried out throughout body and have wide spread effect on various bodily organs. These hormones play an important role from basic body metabolism to mental development, sleep, sex desire, reaction to stress, alertness and secondary sexual characteristics. The endocrine glands are:

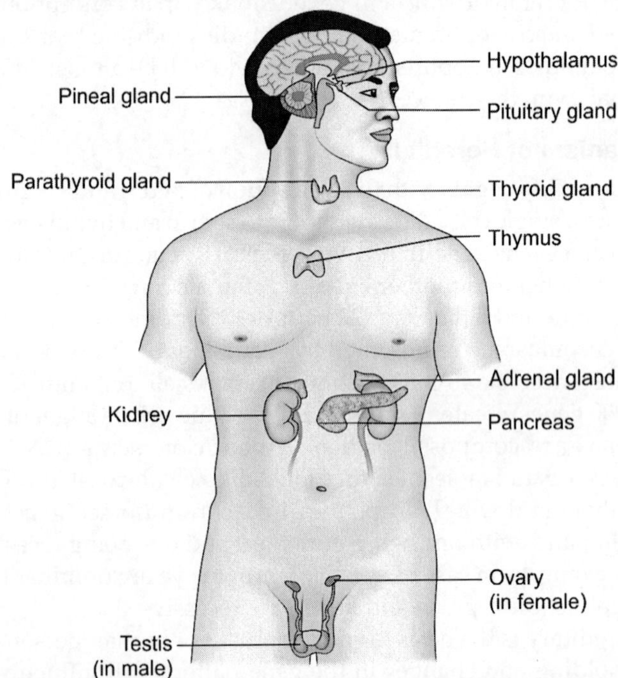

Fig. 2.6: Locations of endocrine glands

- The pituitary gland (master gland)
- Thyroid gland
- Parathyroid
- Adrenals
- Pancreas
- Sex gland (ovary in female and testis in male)

The hormones of endocrine glands have dramatic effects on mood, emotional state, learning, mental and physical development and human personality.

The duct glands release their secretion either into a body cavity or on the surface of the body cavity.

Following are the duct gland in human body:

- Salivary gland
- Sweat gland
- Gastric gland
- Lacrimal gland
- Sex gland

Muscular Control of Behavior

Human behavior is the result of balanced coordination and action of different parts of system. Muscular system plays very important role in expression of thought, feeling and emotions. We move our limbs when we do certain activities like bath, exercise, running, walking, jogging, eating, and dressing, etc. These different activities and behavior are performed with the help of muscle. Muscles are involved in both external and internal body movements. The skeletal muscles enable the individual to make movements by contrasting and relaxing. In contrast, smooth muscle are implied in vital body functions such as elimination, excretion, etc. The coordination and control of muscle determine the precision, speed and strength of movement. Prolonged stimulation, disease, injury or excessive exercise may leads to fatigue due to accumulation of lactic acid in muscle.

Muscle tone refers to the readiness of muscle to contrast. An adequate muscle tone ensures smooth and ready responses. Illness and over exercise may leads to state of hypertonic muscle which may create further problems like problems in walking, digestion, and elimination, etc. An adequate diet, rest and exercise enable to maintain and regains the muscle tone.

Suggested Reading

- Agur A, Dalley AF. Grant's Atlas of Anatomy, 12th edn. Lippincott Williams & Wilkins, 2008.
- Anthikad J. Psychology for Graduate Nurses, 4th edn. New Delhi: Jaypee Brothers Medical Publishers (P) Ltd, 2008.
- Drake RL, Vogl AW, Mitchell AW. Gray's Anatomy for Students, 2nd edn. Churchill Livingstone, 2009.
- Gilroy A, MacPherson B, Ross L, et al. Atlas of Anatomy, 1st edn. Thieme, 2008.
- Hall JE. Guyton and Hall Textbook of Medical Physiology, 12th edn. Elsevier/Saunders, 2010.
- Morgan CT, King RA, Weisz JR, et al. Introduction to Psychology, 7th edn. New Delhi: Tata McGraw Hill Publishing Company Ltd, 2007.
- Plotnik R. Introduction to Psychology, 5th edn. USA: Wadsworth Publishing Company, 1998.
- Raff H, Levitzky M. Medical Physiology: A Systems Approach, 1st edn. McGraw-Hill, 2011.

REVIEW QUESTIONS

SHORT-ESSAY TYPE QUESTIONS

1. Discuss the impact of glands on human behavior.
2. Discuss brain structure and its relation to human behavior.
3. Explain the relationship between heredity and behavior.
4. Discuss psychology of vision sensation.

MULTIPLE CHOICE QUESTIONS

1. Who is known as father of genetics?
   a. Charles Darwin
   b. Gregor Mendel
   c. William James
   d. Sigmund Freud
2. Which part of neuron receives nerve impulses from another neuron?
   a. Axon
   b. Terminal
   c. Dendrites
   d. Cell body

3. The gap between one neuron to another neuron is called:
   a. Synapses
   b. Synaptic cleft
   c. Neurotransmitter
   d. Dendrites
4. Which of the following part of brain responsible for life sustain part of life?
   a. Medulla oblongata
   b. Pons
   c. Cerebellum
   d. Cerebrum
5. Which of the following part of the brain responsible for selective retention?
   a. Medulla oblongata
   b. Pons
   c. Limbic system
   d. Reticular formation
6. Which of the following part of the brain connect left to right hemispheres?
   a. Medulla oblongata
   b. Pons
   c. Corpus callosum
   d. Limbic system
7. Which of the following is the center respiration and heart rate control?
   a. Pons
   b. Cerebrum
   c. Medulla oblongata
   d. Hippocampus
8. Which of the following part of the brain responsible for vision processing?
   a. Frontal
   b. Parietal
   c. Temporal
   d. Occipital
9. Parasympathetic nervous system stimulate following activity:
   a. Heart rate
   b. Blood pressure
   c. Respiratory rate
   d. Gastrointestinal peristalsis
10. 'Flight and Fight' response is mediated by following gland:
    a. Pituitary gland
    b. Adrenal gland
    c. Thyroid gland
    d. Thymus gland

ANSWER KEY

1.	b	2.	c	3.	a	4.	a	5.	d	6.	c	7.	c
8.	d	9.	d	10.	b								

Sensation, Attention and Perception

Chapter 3

INTRODUCTION

Information about the world has to have a way to get into the brain, where it can be used to determine actions and responses. The way into the brain is through the sensory organs and the process of sensation. We get knowledge about ourselves and the world around us through the functioning of our sense organs. Things of these sense organs we see, hear, touch, taste and smell the things around the environment. The impressions received through the sense organs are called sensation.

SENSATION

Sensations are the mind's window to the world that exist around us. Without perception, we would be unable to understand what all those sensations means perception is the process of interpreting the sensations we experience so that we can act upon it.

Definition of Sensation

'A sensation is an elementary cognitive experience' (Jalota)

'Sensations are the first things in the way of consciousness' (James)

'Pure sensation is a psychological myth' (Ward)

In light of the above definition sensation can be best defined sensation as a cognitive process that occurs when special receptors in the sense organs are activated, allowing various forms of outside stimuli become neural signals in the brain.

Nature of Sensation

Through our sense we are presented with an incredibly rich and varied experience of the world, including the aroma of roasting coffee, the texture of fine silk, the taste of good food, the sound of our favorite music, and the sight of glorious sunset. Not all sensations are pleasant and lovely. The senses unflinchingly bring to us an immense range of experiences from the world around us.

The process of converting outside stimuli, such as light into neural activity is called transduction.

The following general characteristics are present in every sensation through light on nature of a particular sensation:

- **Quality:** Every sensation has some quality. For example, a color may be green, red or yellow. A taste may be bitter, sour or sweet, a sound may be pleasant or intolerable. Quality may be studied under two subheadings.
- **Kind:** Sensations differ in quality on account of different kinds. Sensations of color, sound, tastes, smells, heats and cold differ from one another quality. They have different sense organs. They are produced by different kind of stimuli.
- **Modality:** Sensation belong to same sense organ also differ from one another. Visual sensation differs among themselves according to nature of stimuli such as light –blue, green, red and yellow. There even more exact difference exists in quality. There are innumerable shades of blue, green, red and yellow light.
- **Intensity or quantity:** Every sensation has some intensity and it is noticed because of that intensity. For example, the buzzing sound of a mosquito is not heard from a yard distance, it must be strong enough to get noticed. The intensity of light from 20 candles is stronger than 10 candles. Taste also may be weak or strong.
- **Duration or potensity:** Every sensation lasts for a certain length of time, however small it may be. Sensation may be last longer or transitory in nature.
- **Extensity:** Extensity refer to extension in space or space aspect. It is variably known as volume, diffusion, massiveness, or spread out-ness. Extensity not true for all types of sensations. Look at the moon than on star. You have two visual sensations. The whiteness of a classroom wall is more extensive than the whiteness of the paper.
- **Clarity:** Every sensation has clarity. The sensation which is long-lasting becomes more clear than the sensation of transitory sensation.
- **Local sign:** Sensations differ from one another in local sign. If we touch the skin of different body surface area, i.e. palm, nose, ear, check and hips with applying equal pressure for the same duration, touch will differ from one touch to another due to special attributes of the different kind of surface touched. We

have several sense organs. Fundamentals of human senses are described in Table 3.1.

Table 3.1: Fundamentals of human senses

Sense	Stimulus	Sense organ	Sensation
Sight	Light waves	Eye	Colors, patterns, textures
Hearing	Sound waves	Ear	Noise, tones, music
Skin sensation	External touch	Skin	Touch, cold, warmth, pain
Smell	Volatile materials	Nose	Odors
Taste	Soluble materials	Tongue	Sweet, salty, bitter

- **Sensory receptors:** The sensory receptors are specialized forms of neurons, the cells that make-up the nervous system. Instead of receiving neurotransmitter from other cells, there receptor cells are stimulated by different kind of energy for example, the receptors in eye by light, whereas the receptors in ear are stimulated by sound. Touch receptors stimulated by pressure and temperature, and the taste receptors are triggered by chemical substances.

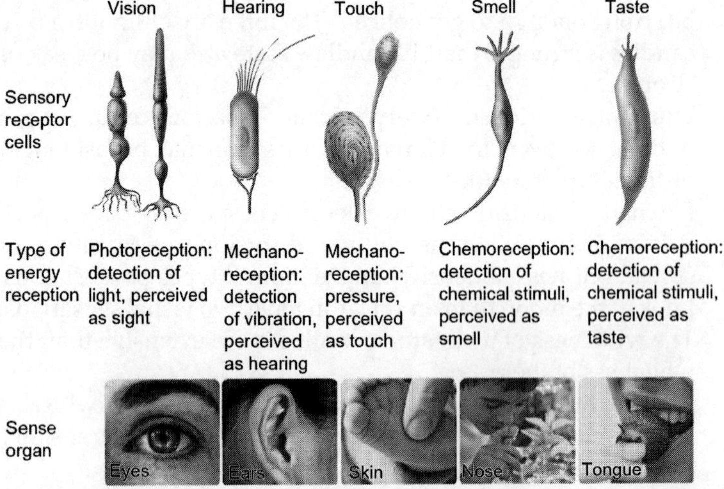

Fig. 3.1: Human sense organs, energy stimuli and sensory receptors

- **Absolute threshold:** E Weber (1795-1878) gave the concept of difference threshold or just noticeable difference (JND). A JND is the smallest difference between two stimuli, i.e. detectable

50% of the time. Later Gustav Fechner (1801–1887) expanded the concept of Weber and given gave concept of *absolute threshold*. An absolute threshold is the lowest level of stimulation that a person can consciously detect 50 percent of time stimulation is present. For example, in a very quiet room and normal hearing, how far way can you hear the tick of watch on half of the trials?

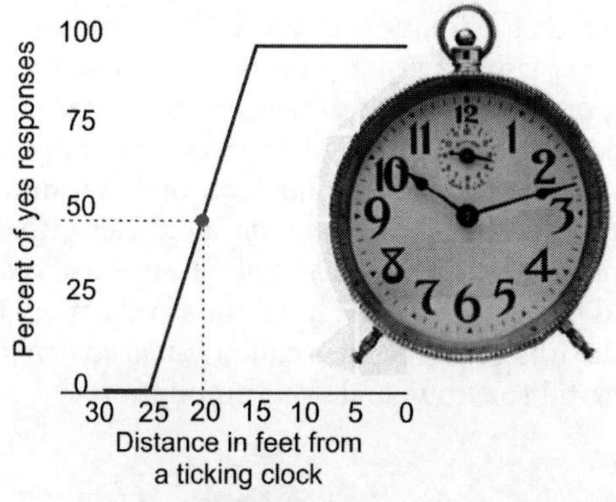

Fig. 3.2: Measuring absolute threshold

Table 3.2: Examples of measuring absolute threshold

Sight	A candle flame at 30 miles on a clear, dark night
Hearing	The tick of a watch 20 feet away in a quiet room
Smell	One drop of perfume diffused throughout a three room apartment
Taste	A teaspoon of sugar in 2 gallons of water
Touch	A bee's wing falling on the cheek from 1 centimeter above

We have several sense organs; let us briefly discuss anatomy of these sense organs.

EYE

The structures of the eye play a vital role in both collecting and focusing of light so we can see clearly. The surface of the eye is covered in a clear membrane called the cornea. The cornea not only protects the eye but also is the structure that focuses most of the light coming into the eye. The cornea has a fixed structure, like a camera that has no option to adjust the focus. However, this curvature can be changed somewhat through vision improving techniques that change the shape of cornea. For example, *laser assisted in-situ keratomileusis (LASIK)* and *photorefractive keratectomy (PRK)*.

The next visual layer is a clear, watery fluid called the aqueous humor. This fluid is continually replenished and supplies nourishment to the eye. The light from the visual image into enters the interior of the eye through a hole, called pupil, in a round muscle called the iris (the colored part of the eye). The iris is responsible for changing the size of the pupil to focus the image on retina. Behind the iris, is another clear structure called the lens. The lens also helps to focus the image on retina. The variation in thickness allows the lens to protect a sharp image on retina.

Once light cross the lens, it passes through a large, open space filled with a clear jelly like fluid called the *vitreous humor*. The nature and function of this fluid is similar to aqueous humor. The final stop for light within the eye is the *retina,* a light sensitive area at the back of the eye opening called *blind spot*. The optic nerve leave from blind spot and blind spot do not have rods and cones. The process of adjusting the image on retina is called *visual accommodation*. Eye lenses play a vital role in visual accommodation.

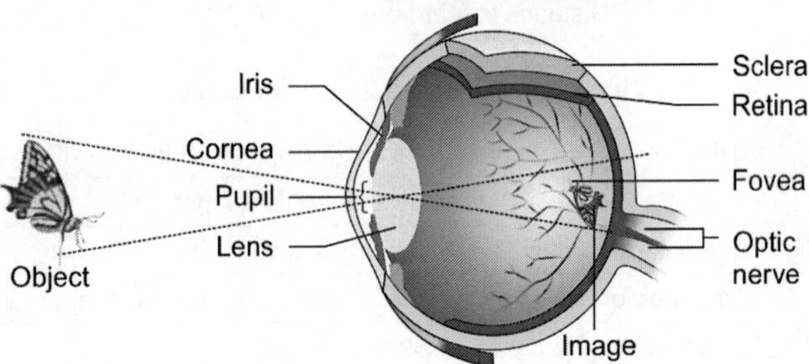

Fig. 3.3: Structure of an eye

Physiology of Vision

The eye is the special sense organ for the sensation of light. Light waves are the external stimuli. The proper organ is the retina with in the eye ball. Light wave act upon the retina and the sensation is carried out to the brain by optic nerve and we perceive the image. The retina is very sensitive to light and is made up of rods and cones. The rod and cones in the retina are the proper receptors in sensations. Visual sensations are of two types:

1. **Sensation of brightness:** White, black, gray refer to sensation of brightness regarded as the most primitive and earliest sensations.
2. **Sensation of color:** Red, yellow, green and blue are primary. Color blind people do not feel these sensations.

EAR

The ear is the sense organ for hearing. The stimulus consists in vibration of the air. An auditory sensation is the response of the ear to air vibrations. Usually the local symbol is absent in auditory sensation in which the power of discrimination is high.

Anatomy

The ear is a series of structure and divided into three parts:

1. **External ear:** The pinna is the visible, external part of the ear that serve as a kind of concentrator, funneling the sound wave from outside into auditory canal, a short tunnel that run down to the tympanic membrane. When sound waves hit the ear drum, they cause three tiny bones in the middle ear to vibrate.
2. **Middle ear:** It consists three small bones, hammer, anvil, and stirrup. These are known as *malleus*, *incus* and *stapes*. Stapes is the smallest bone of human body. The main function of these three bones is to amplify the vibration from the eardrum.
3. **Inner ear:** The membrane of inner ear is called *oval window*. The inner ear has a snail shaped in structure called *cochlea*. Vibration in oval window leads to vibration in fluid in the cochlea. This fluid surround a membrane running through middle of cochlea called *basilar membrane*.

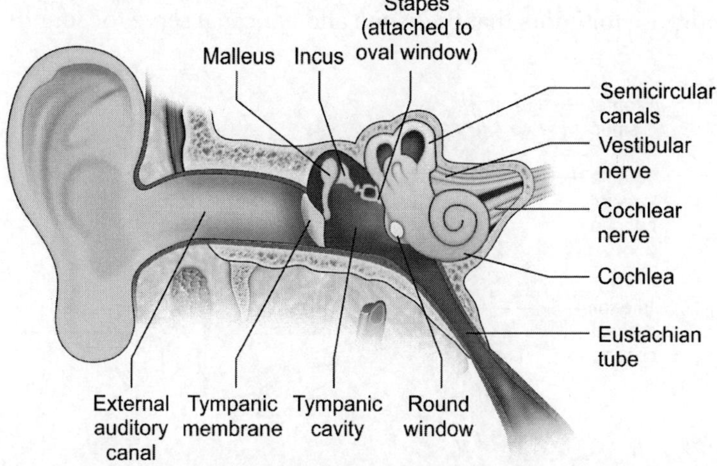

Fig. 3.4: Structure of an ear

The basilar membrane is the resting place of *organ of Corti,* which contains receptor cells of the sense of hearing, called *hair cells.* When these hair cells bent up against the other membrane, it causes them to send a neural massage through the *auditory nerve* in to the brain, where auditory cortex will interrupt the sounds and we hear. Elements of auditory sensations are:

- **Pitch:** It is highness or lowness of sound. It depends upon the rate or frequency of air vibration. The greater the vibration, the higher is the pitch.
- **Timber:** Timber is the peculiar quality of a tone produced musical instrument. Timber depends upon the quality of air wave.
- **Harmony:** Certain tones fuse with one another and produce an aggregate effect in consciousness. This is called harmony or consonance.
- **Discord:** Some tone refuse to fuse and are harsh called discordant in their effect on our mind.

NOSE (SENSATION OF SMELL)

Nose is the special sensory organ for sensation of smell or odor. The stimuli for olfaction are in the form of sebaceous substance, vapor, and small particles. There is mechanical chemical reaction between the stimulus and the sense organ. This is called olfaction or the olfactory sense. The outer part of the nose serve the same purpose for odors that the pinna and ear canal serve for sounds.

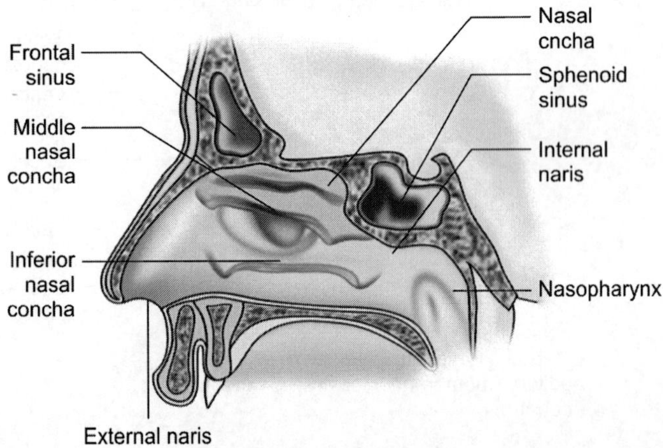

Fig. 3.5: Structure of nose

The part of the olfactory system that transduces odors-turns odors into signals the brain can understand is allocated at the roof of the nasal passages. Olfactory receptors cells each have about to a dozen little 'hairs', called *cilia* that project into the cavity. Like taste buds they send signals to the brain and we feel odor.

TONGUE (SENSATION OF TASTE)

The sense organ of the sensation of the taste is the tongue. Taste is also contributed by soft palate but the tongue is the main organ of sense. The receptors for the sensation of taste are called taste buds. These are found in the papillae of the tongue and are widely distributed in the epithelium of the tongue, soft palate, pharynx and epiglottis. The tongue of an adult nearly contains 10,000 taste buds. Each bud is a oval structure which consists of three kinds of epithelial cells. They are the gustatory receptor cells, supporting cells and the basal cells.

Each taste bud contains about forty taste receptor cells, that extend into a tiny opening in the epithelium of the taste bud, called a taste pore. Taste buds are found in elevation, of the tongue called papillae. They are circumvallate papillae, fungifrom and Filiform papillae. Each taste bud has about 20 receptors and acts like a neuron at synapse site.

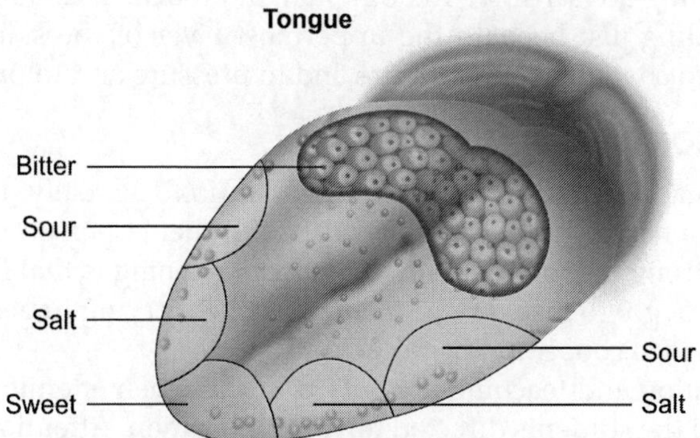

Fig. 3.6: Structure of tongue (placement of taste buds)

SKIN

This is the largest organ of human body. Skin serves many purposes; sensation of touch, temperature, cold, heat regulation, immunity maintenance, and keeping bodily fluid in and germs out.

There are about half dozen of different receptors in the skin. Different receptors respond in different sensation. For example, *Pacinian corpuscles* are just beneath the skin and respond to change in pressure.

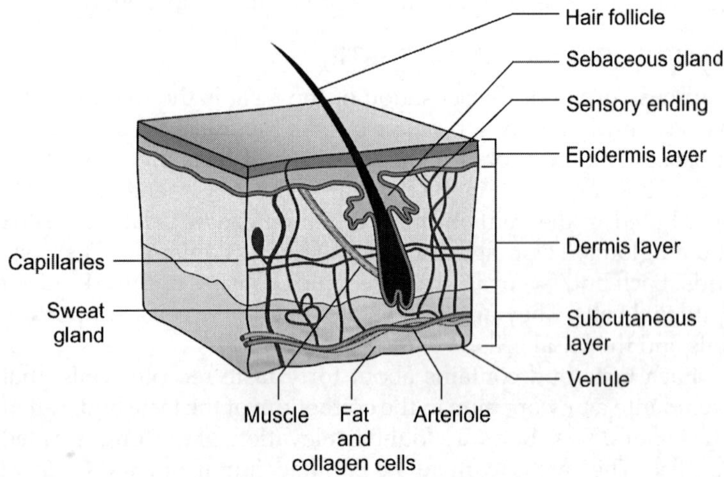

Fig. 3.7: Structure of skin

There are nerves ending wrap around the hair follicles. These nerve ending are sensitive to both pain and touch. There are free nerve ending just beneath the uppermost layer of the skin that respond to change in temperature and to pressure and to pain.

ATTENTION

When a teacher say, 'Please give your attention', he really means, 'please attend to what I am going to say'. When a person is said to have strong power of attention, the real meaning is that he can attend strongly to his work or to an object he is trying to observe. To attend is to concentrate your activity.

Education and teaching are only possible when attention and interest of the students directed towards education. Attention and interest plays vital role in learning and teaching process.

Nature of Attention

Definition and Meaning of Attention

'Attention is the process of getting an object of thought clearly before the mind' (Ross)

'Attention is concentration of mind'

(Woodworth and Schlosberg)

'Attention is the selective act of consciousness'

(Rex and Knight)

'Attention is the tendency to dwell on an object so as to understand it theoretically and practically' (Stout)

In the light of above definition it can be concluded that attention is a selective process in which only one response is given out of various simultaneous stimuli.

Characteristics of Attention

The following are the important characteristics:

- **Selectivity:** Attention is selective activity of the mind. At a given moment many stimuli act upon the sense organ but only few will be selected by the sense organs.
- **Shifting:** Attention is always shifting rapidly. Attention to any single object cannot last for very long time and within few seconds it will shift to another object. It rises and falls and shifts from one object to another. For example, while reading a book our attention shift from one word to another and sometimes to external environment.
- **Purposeful:** Attention is purposeful in nature. The objects or things which are directed are related to us will be selected more attentive.
- **Effortful:** Attention needs both physical and mental energy. You can also notice it that in case you feel tired or fatigue, your attention to lecture will be reduced.
- **Aspect of mental activity:** Attention implies all the three kinds of mental activity, i.e cognitive, conative and affective.
- **Narrow scope:** Attention is limited to only few things at a single time. We cannot attend so many objects at a time.
- **Exploratory in nature:** Attention is exploratory in nature. When we attend new object, we tend to explore its different qualities and attributes.
- **Attention is positive and negative in nature:** When you attend certain things your mind will focus on certain parts of the things (positive things) and ignore certain part of the things (negative aspects).

Types of Attention

- **Active attention:** Active attention is characterized by presence of will, interest and mental effort of an individual. Active attention depends on our choice. We can also say that active attention depends on our interest to attend the things.
- **Passive attention:** Passive attention is the absence of features of active attention (will, interest and mental effort). Sometimes, it is also known as spontaneous attention. For example, paying attention to band music while studying.
- **Involuntary attention:** This attention is against the will and mental activity of subject. For example, while preparing for exam you have to attend sudden marriage party noise outside.
- **Immediate attention:** Attention is immediate when object is interesting in itself. For example, suddenly paying attention to the song of interest.
- **Sensory attention:** Sensory attention is practical and empirical attention. For example, paying attention to objects like sofa, TV and toys at home.
- **Ideational attention:** Ideational attention is attention to thought, images, words of others like image of your loved teacher, your loving things like pen, watch, etc.

Importance of Attention

Attention is most basic prerequisite for classroom teaching. It helps teaching learning in following ways:

- **Teaching and learning:** Attention is the most basic prerequisite for teaching and learning in the classroom. Attention only makes learning and teaching effective and efficient.
- **Aid to memory:** Attention is valuable aid to memory. Material learned with full attention will remain last longer in our memory.
- **Acquisition of skills:** Paying strong attention helps to learn skills and competency. Learning all skills depend upon attention.
- **Speed of learning:** Attention improve the speed of learning and helps to learn quickly.
- **Success and achievement:** It has seen that paying attentions learning material leads to success and good achievement in all fields.

Factors Influencing Attention

Factors or conditions affecting attention are broadly classified under following domains:

- **Objective (environmental) factors:** These are the factors which are related to object or environment in which object is present. Objective factors are as follows:
  - **Intensity:** A strong stimulus attract our attention more quickly than the weak one. For example, a loud sound, bright light or intense pain can get attention very quickly than others. Some things like bright color, hot tastes and strong odor attract our attention more quickly.
  - **Size of stimuli (object):** A bigger size object captures attention more easily than a smaller one. For example, a bigger size of hording or advertisement at roadside or in newspaper easily attracts our attention. Hence, circus and cinema owners use big posters to catch the attention of people.
  - **Novelty:** New object easily attract our attention. New fashion, new sound, new equipments and newly designed program draw attention easily.
  - **Change:** Change in the law of nature. Change in the stimulus is likely to draw attention more easily. For example, new arousal sound in classroom or office will draw attention quickly than tickling sound of a clock.
  - **Contrast:** A contrast object catch the attention more quickly than a dull or ordinary color object. For example, a black ship in hundreds of white ship, a black women dancing on dance floor among white women.
  - **Strangeness:** Uncommon or strange stimuli draw attention more easily than routine one. For example, a western dressing style man and woman among Indian dressed population are easily attended.
  - **Repetition of stimuli:** It has been suggested that repeated stimuli have shorter subjective duration than novel items, perhaps because of a reduction in the neural response to repeated presentation of the same subject and reduced the attention.
  - **Movements:** A moving object draw attention than a steady one. For example, in railway platform, we draw attention

quickly to moving train. Most of the advertisers try to capture the attention of people through moving electric lights.

- **Striking or unusual quality:** An object possessing unusual quality is more likely to draw our attention. A teacher with outstanding communication, novel ideas can attract more easily the attention of the students.

- **Subjective factors:** Subjective factors related to individual. These factors may be related to physical or mental aspects of an individual.
  - **Interest:** Interest is the most basic requirement for attention. Interest is the most powerful dictator of attention. Usually we attend the object in which we are interested. For example, a boy interested in world wrestling entertainment (WWE) will be more attentive to watch WWE than other sports at television.
  - **Instincts:** Instincts are 'prime movers' of our behavior, so the things which appeal to instincts attract our attention. For example, when we hungry; we attract to food, when we are thirsty; we attract to water, etc.
  - **Emotions:** Emotions are said to be 'internal motivations' of attention. Joy, sorrow, love, hate all are emotions. In case of happiness, we attend bright aspects of life like rocking songs and in case of sadness; we attract so sadistic phenomena like listening sad songs, etc.
  - **Temperament:** People with different temperament attend different objects. For example, an extroverted personality attracts to attend more social things than introverted one.
  - **Habits:** Habit is a great incentive in attention. A person habitual of certain things will easily attract to that particular things. For example, a smoker to smoking and an alcoholic to drink or alcohol related products. On the other hand a person with habit of reading books will attract to books or magazine more easily.
  - **Mental set:** Mental set is an important factor of drawing attention. A person always attends to those objects towards which his mind is set. For example, a person who invited a friend to come at 5 pm will attract to door with a small knock at 5 pm.

- **Physiological factors:** Fatigue and illness destroy attention and interest. Chronic fatigue and illness may decrease attention span to eve most interesting thing. Freshness is conducive to attention. A healthy physical and mental set can attend to something for longer time.

- **Social factors:** Society play an important role in establishing the object of our attention. Our family, playmates, neighborhood, class fellow and society to determine our attention at large. Our likings, disliking, attitude, all are influenced by social environment, prejudice, social taboos that determine our interest and attention in certain things.

PERCEPTION

Human activities belong to knowing, feelings and willing. Perception belongs primarily to knowing. It is a cognitive process. The objects are presented to us thorough the medium of sensation. Sensations are essential to perception. Thus, perception means knowledge of object which comes through sensation. Hence perception = sensation + meaning.

Definition

'Perception is that mental process by which we get knowledge of objective facts' (Jalota)

'The process of interpretation of sensation according to experiences is known as perception' (Ryburn)

'Perception is the process of getting to know objects and objective facts by the use of senses' (Woodworth)

'Perception is the process of obtaining knowledge of external object and events by means of senses' (Stagner)

'Perception is an individual awareness aspect or behavior; for it is the way each person process the raw data he/she receives from the environment in to meaningful patterns.' (Silverman)

So, on the basis of above definition we can say that perception is a conative, complex and cognitive process aroused by stimulation of sense organ. It gives us knowledge of things in the external world which can be analyzed by perception.

NATURE AND CHARACTERISTICS OF PERCEPTION

- **Perception is cognitive:** Perception is a cognitive process. Cognition means knowledge. The cognition of knowledge of object is called perception. It is the process of obtaining knowledge of external world, i.e. object, events and facts by the use of senses.

- **Perception based on sensation:** Perception means knowledge of object which through sensation. Without sensation perception is not possible. Perception involves sensation. It is a process of interpreting or giving meaning to sensation.
- **Perception involves memory and thought:** Perception is concerned with cognition and recognition of the things. Hence, it involves memory and a spontaneous and perhaps unconscious inference or thought activity over and above the sensation. That why it is sometimes said perception = sensation + thought.
- **Perception is selective:** Perception is highly selective. Many stimuli act on our sense organs but only very few or selected stimuli sensitize the organ. Perception is ultimately based on the principle of pick and chooses. Selection of perception depends on many things like habit, interest, like, dislike, sentiments, needs, motives and readiness etc.
- **Perception is preventative and representative:** Perception is presentative as well as representative in nature. It influence by external stimuli (presentative) and it involves memory and imagination (representative).
- **Perception is synthetic experience:** Perception is synthetic in terms of combination of new and the old experiences.
- **Perception is attentive:** Without attention perception is not possible. Attention is mandatory for clear and distinct perception.
- **Perception is accompanied by feeling and action:** Perception is always accompanied by feelings and actions. We perceive rose by touching and feel it by fragrance likewise a runner perceive the road by his muscular action and feel it endurance. So perception is related to feelings and actions.
- **Figure and ground in perception:** Figure and ground refers to the most basic and element necessity of perceptual structure. We perceive an object as figure in ground. For example, we perceive the moon in sky. Her moon is the figure and sky is the ground. We perceive a picture on wall, here picture is figure and wall is ground. This tendency for the perceptual field is to divide the perceptual field in primacy (important) and secondary (unimportant) is referred as figure ground theory of perception

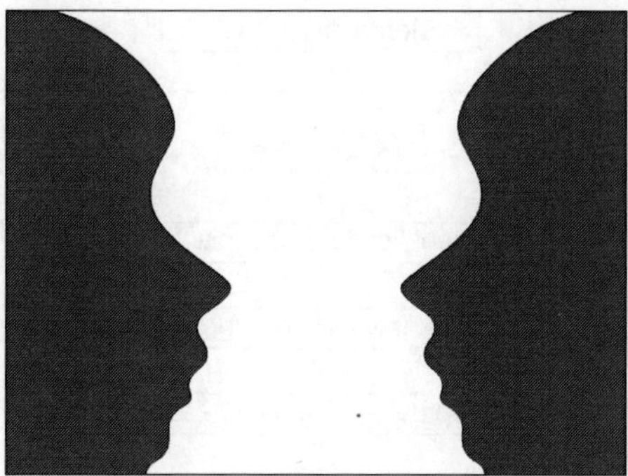

Fig. 3.8: Figure and ground phenomena

Rubin concluded figure and ground theory as below:

- Figure has to form where ground is relatively formless. If the ground has to form qualities, it appears to have a weaker and definite contour.
- Figure has 'thing like' qualities, whereas ground appears as more homogenous and unformed material.
- Figure appears to be nearer to the observer than does the ground. The ground appears to extend and unbroken behind the figure.
- The figure is more easily identified and named then ground
- The color of the figure is more impressive
- The figure is connected with meaning, feelings and aesthetic value than is the ground.

Rubin also noted that when he presented the same nonsense form a second time, there was often a reversal of figure and ground. What had been figure became ground and what had been ground became figure. The above is one of the Rubin's figures. It is the twin and vase example as one looks at it, one sees the vase as figure and the black portion as the ground; then the organization reverses; so that the black position is seen as the twin looking at one another, and the white area becomes the ground.

The conditions that favor the organization of parts to figure or whole are their nearness, similarity, continuity, inclusiveness, familiarity and person's set of readiness.

- **Perception is a complex phenomenon:** Perception is very deep and complex phenomena involving many processes like receptors process, unification, symbolization and affection, etc.

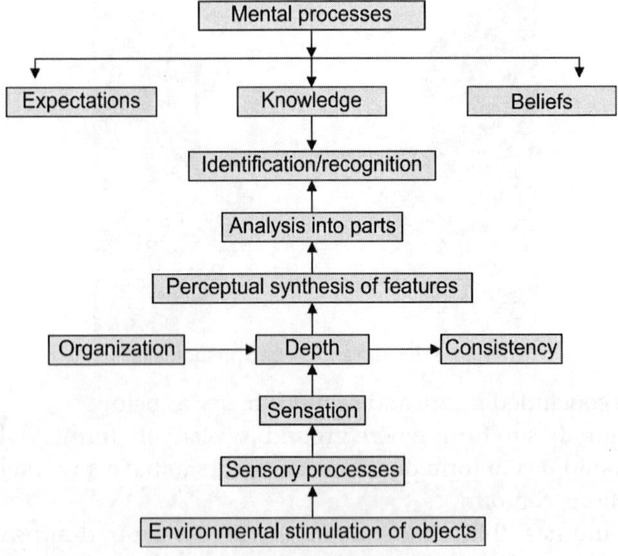

Fig. 3.9: Process of perception

- **Perception is an process:** It is essentially a process rather than being a product or outcomes or some psychological phenomena.
- **Perception is an individualized process:** It is highly individualized psychological process that helps an organism in organizing and interpreting the complex pattern of sensory stimuli for giving them the necessary meaning to initiate his/her behavioral responses.

Difference between Sensation and Perception

Some of the main differences are explained here:

- **Simple versus complex phenomena:** Sensation is a simple or elementary process while perception is complex mental process. Perception involves much beside sensation. In perception, we interpret sensation, i.e. process of interpretation. Memory, though also play equal role in process of interpretation.
- **Passive versus active:** Perception is active process as compare to passive sensation. In sensation, our mind merely receives impression from the external stimulus while in perception it only receives but also contributes something from its past experiences.

- **Abstract vs concrete:** Sensation is the abstraction of the mind or a result of analysis while perception is an actual, concrete experience of mind.
- **Sensible qualities vs objects:** Sensation is always a sensation of sensible qualities; while perception is always a perception of an object.
- **Primary vs secondary:** Sensation is primary while perception is secondary. Sensation is primary and first in the sequence of time while perception is secondary.
- **Awareness vs apperception:** Sensation is merely an awareness of something while perception implies apperception.
- **New vs mixed experiences:** In sensation, all knowledge is free from past experiences and fresh while in perception past experiences does matter.
- **Physiological vs psychological:** Sensation are of physiological process and body related while perception is more of psychological in nature and related to mind.
- **Mechanical vs purposeful:** Sensation is blind, automatic and mechanical process. Perception is meaningful and purposeful in nature.
- **Vague vs definite:** Sensation is dim and vague process. It only become clear and definite when it is converted into a perception.

FACTORS INFLUENCING PERCEPTION

There are many factors that may influence perception; broadly, these factors are classified under the following headings:

- Gestalt law of organization
- Objective (environmental) factors
- Subjective factors
- Social factors

Gestalt Law of Organization: One important characteristics of the perceived world is that it is full of shapes, forms or pattern, which are quiet stable and often unchanging. According to Gestalt psychologists the perceptual world cannot think off a sample of sum total sensory input. There are organization tendencies with a person which act as a sensory data to produce the world of experience. Gestalt law of organization emphasizes the relative importance of perceiving while object forms and proposed a number of principles or laws of how we organize objects:

- **Law of Figure and Ground** (see in factors)
- **Principle of Contour:** The separation of object from the general background in visual perception is possible only because of the perceptual principle known as *contour.* For example, if we look at the homogenous background, unfilled with any shades, lights or object (i.e. clear sky), we can see no contour. But, if same ground is filled with bright and dark lights we can easily see contour formation. A contour can be defined as line of demarcation perceived by an observer whenever there is a marked difference between the brightness or color in one part of the visual field and other. However, contour can sometimes be seen without the difference in brightness in the perceptual field and this type of contour recalled *subjective contour.*
- **Principle of Closure:** We should also bear in mind that the perception of object which we see in our perceptual field is much more complete than the sensory stimulation received by us from an object. Our perception may supply elements which are not be found in our sensory data till we perceive a thing as a meaningful whole. Thus, an incomplete drawing of circle or triangles can be perceived as circle or triangle. In other words, it can be perceived as a whole rather than art. This tendency to fill the gap perceptually when a stimulus is incomplete is known as *law of fragrance* or *law of closure.*

Fig. 3.10: Principle of closure

- **Principle of Grouping:** The other organizing tendency in our perception is known as grouping when our perceptual field is filling up with a number of stimuli and organizing tendencies try to bring some order in it by grouping the object in the visual field, into some pattern or shape. But, it is also true that this type of grouping is not at all conscious effort from a person but it is a tendency in the brain and senses to see things or grouped it in some way. Perceptual grouping takes place according to some basic principles or laws:

- **Law of Proximity (Nearness):** Stimuli which are close together in space and time tend to be perceived together. More the proximity, better the perception.
  - For example, together that are easily flies combined with group

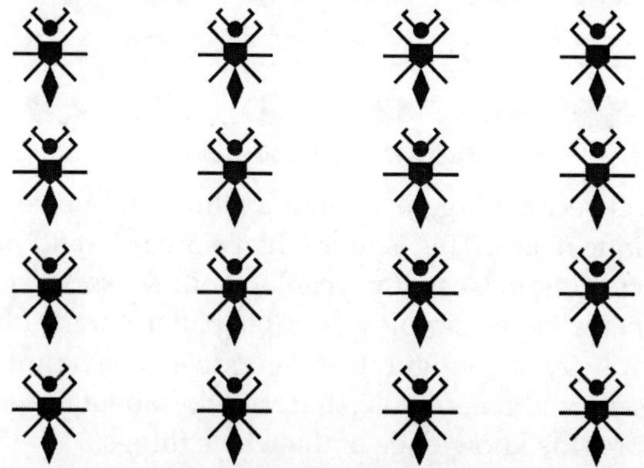

Fig. 3.11: Principle of proximity (nearness)

  - When we look at star at night, we group stars as close to one another in a pattern and perceives them as a whole. We perceive them into a triangle, a circle or into a straight line.

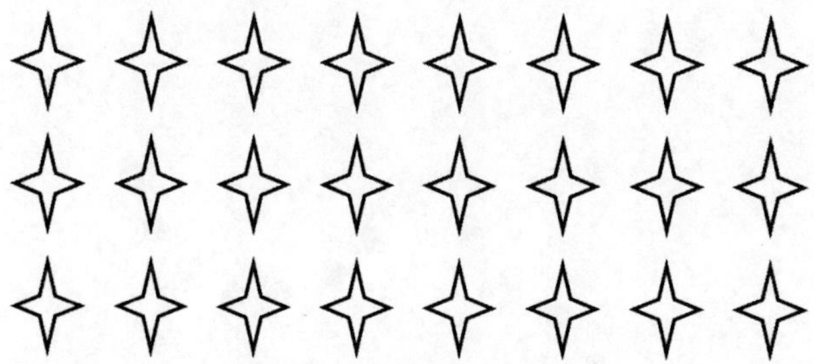

Fig. 3.12: Principle of closure

- **Law of Similarity:** Stimuli which are similar tend to be perceived as forming a group. A collection of data naturally breaks up into two combinations when dots are of two steps:
- **Law of Symmetry:** Symmetry influences our perception. When we place some object in order of symmetry, the various

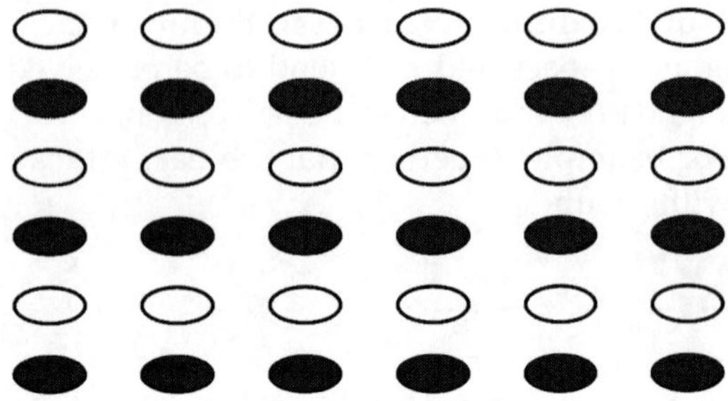

Fig. 3.13: Law of similarity

parts become organized into a whole and perceives as an unique object. This is more than similarity and proximity. According to Gestalt psychology our sensory organs tend to perceive the simplest possible pattern of the object. The simplicity or configurational goodness of a figure is said to observe the general rule, the formation about the part is able to provide knowledge of the whole things.

- **Law of Adaptability:** When we are adapted to any object or event we perceive the object in a whole manner. It means adaptability facilitates the perceptual process.
- **Law of Continuity/Closure:** Perception of many objective facts is determined by the principle of continuity. Mind the following two given examples:

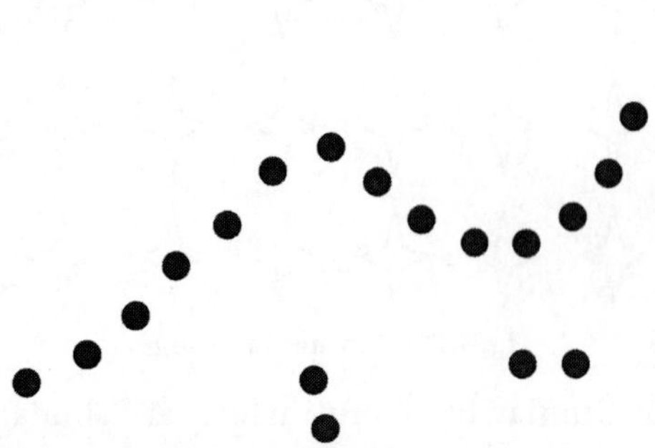

Fig. 3.14: Law of continuity

In case of group A. For example, the tendency of the number 11 is perceived after 9 but in case of group B this is not possible.

- **Law of Completeness:** Completeness is a factor of advantage in perception. A group which includes all parts in it has an advantage over what leaves some parts outside it.

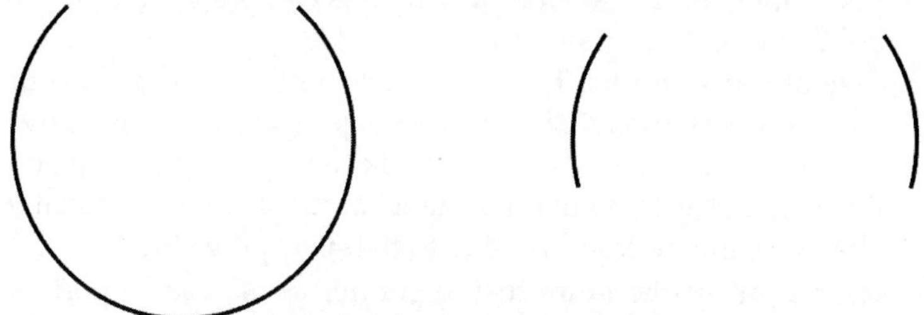

Fig. 3.15: Law of completeness

- **Law of Movement:** A moving object perceived more quickly than stationary one. For example, moving train or high speeds motor bike.
- **Law of Change:** Change is the basic of perception. Change in place, events and things facilitate our perception. Homogeneous things are not quickly and effectively perceived as new or changed one.
- **Low of Prägnanz (whole form):** We tend to perceive stimulus as good form. Good forms tend to be symmetrical, balanced and complete.

Objective factors: These factors are also known as external factors or factors related to the features of stimuli that govern attention. These factors are grouped under five major heads: prepotency, change, size, repetition and movement.

1. **Prepotency:** Some stimuli are highly propnent to draw our attention. In the process of attention, the more intense stimuli attract more attention, in terms of intense color, sound, smell, flower, pressure, etc. Prepotency depends not only on the intense stimulus but also the past experience. The familiar stimulus is more intense to draw our attention to rather than unfamiliar stimuli. For example, when you are seeing a list of names, a close friend's name or names of close relatives will grasp your attention faster than other names.
2. **Change in stimulus:** Human attention is very intense to unusual stimuli in the environment, as the usual stimuli are less responsive in the phenomenon of sensory adaption. Any sudden

change in the stimulus grasps attention faster than other usual objects. For example, while reading newspaper, our attention is attracted by reverse or bold letter. While reading the previous point, most of the time our attention is easily attracted by the bold letter in the paragraph.

3. **Size of the stimulus:** The size of the stimulus also draws our attention very easily. The big size objects are more attractive than the small ones. When we walk through a market place, the bigger objects or advertisement boards are more frequently observed and noticed. It is due to the size of the objects.
4. **Repetition of the stimulus:** Repetition is also an important determinant of attracting one's attention. For example, words mispronounced once in a while will not be noticed or ignored, but if that happens frequently, the mistakes will be noticed very easily. A week stimulus also becomes effective, if it is repeated again and again.
5. **Movement of the stimulus:** We are more sensitive to moving object than a still object in the environment. For example, in an advertisement a moving sign board will be more attractive than a still board.

Subjective factors: These factors are related to internal characteristics of a person. Because of individual differences subjects may differ in perception.

- **Readiness:** Readiness at particular moment is a factor of advantage in perception. If someone ready to see or hear something, he can easily perceive it clearly.
- **Interest:** Perception is influenced by interest of an individual. Interest is powerful predictor of attention and perception. Interest and perception go side by side. It is interest which inspires perception.
- **Habit:** Habit is a great incentive in perception. Habit is based on past experiences. If we are habituated to a particular thing, our perception is immediately attracted by it.
- **Attitude:** Perception is determined by our own attitude. Attitude has been called central factors which guide one is perception of external object and things. For example, in case of we have unfavorable attitude to smoking, the person with smoking also perceived dejected or reduced.

- **Sentiment:** Perception also determined by our sentiment. Objects which are connected with sentiments attract our perception easily. For example, the person who is sentimental to old songs will attract to sound of old songs very quickly.
- **Past experiences:** Good and bitter experiences also influence the perception. For example, a child bitten by dog in childhood will perceive all dogs dangerous.
- **Mental set:** Mental set refers to psychological preparedness of mind to perceive something. For example, if you have invited someone to come at 4 pm then a single knock will quickly draw you to perceive your friend.

Social Factors: Social factors also determine our perception. Our perception is also influenced by our family, classmates, society rituals, neighbor and playmates at large. Our liking, disliking, habit, interest, and attitude all our largely influenced by social environment. A child brought up in a non-vegetarian family delight in the signals of it and enjoys it but on the other hand a child brought up a vegetarian family may perceive it disgusting.

Errors in Perception

Errors in perception are common. Errors in perception may be temporary or permanent. Perception errors may be due to defect in sense organ or environmental influences. Following types of perceptual errors are common: *Illusion and hallucination.*

Illusion

An illusion is a wrong perception. It is wrong or misinterpretation of the object. There are some external stimuli and they wrongly interpreted. For example, a rope for snake, and a patch of moonlight for a ghost, etc.

Definition of illusion

'Illusions are confused or misinterpreted perception'

(Murphy)

'An illusion consists in getting a false impression of the objective facts that are presented to the senses' (Woodworth)

Types of illusion

Illusions arise from all kinds of sensation but the most common are those which rise in connection with sight. They are called optical illusion which are of the following types:

- **Form of Illusion:** The height of a square looks greater than its breadth

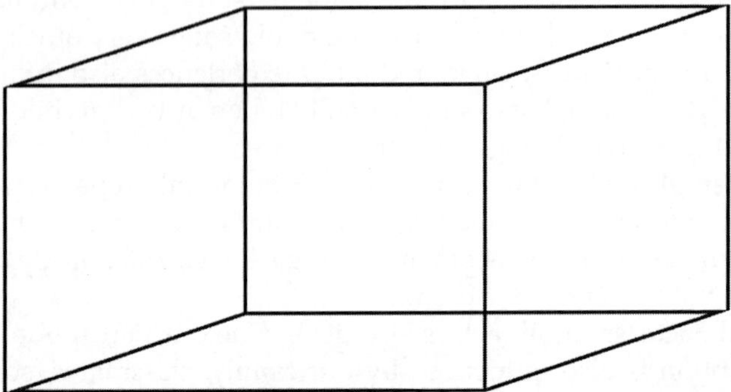

Fig. 3.16: Form of illusion

- **Size of Illusion:** The following figures gives very good example. For example, Muller layer illusion; AB looks longer than CD through they are of the same size.

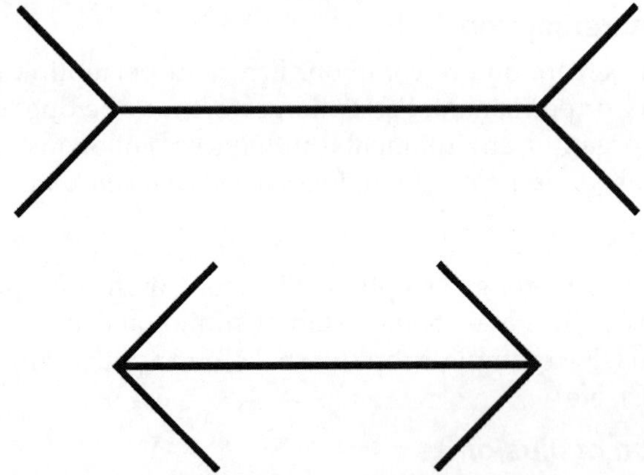

Fig. 3.17: Muller-Lyer illusion

- **Direction of Illusion:** The seen direction of two parallel rails is illusory. They seem to meet at a certain point, though we know that they do not. In the following figures the vertical lines appear to be inclined to one another, through in reality they are parallel. Similarity in the following examples the hospital lines appear to be bent due to the effect of lines that intersect them.

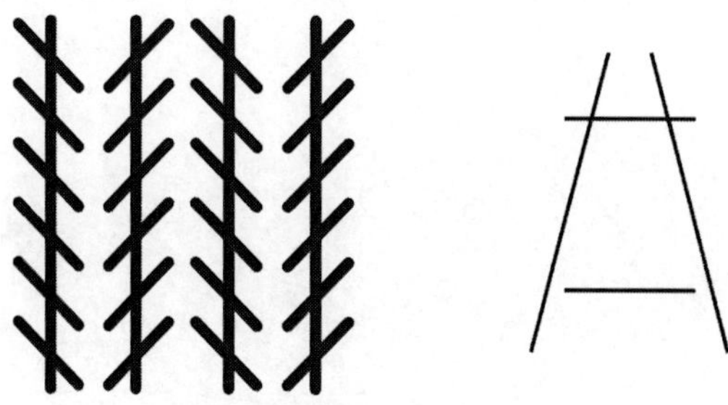

Fig. 3.18: Illusion of direction

- **Illusion of movement:** Sometimes the objects which are at rest seems to be moving, while those are moving seem to be at rest. For example, when we travel in a fast moving train, the tress and houses nearby appear to move in the opposite direction, though they do not really move. This illusion is due to the fast movement of the train.
- **Illusion of distance:** The deceptive nearness of the distant mountain in a clear atmosphere is an example of this illusion. To a pediatrician, the town looks near, through these are all the fields and the woods, and quite number of poles along the railway lines to pass, it may be a good 5 km away.

Causes of Illusion

There could be many factors and conditions related to illusion in a normal human being. Some of common distortions are given here:

- **Defect of sense organs:** Sometimes illusion take lace due to defect of our sense organs. For example, a person suffering from jaundice may perceive while object as yellow. Everything appe rs to be pale to him. A color blind person may perceive color wrongly.
- **Limitations of sense organ:** Our sense organs have their natural power of sensation and perception. Their natural power is limited. Hence, sometime they give us false information about the external world. For example, eye is limited in perception of objects which are too small or too far away. Similarly, ear cannot hear sound which are very low or loud.
- **Peculiarity of sense organs:** Many illusions take place due to peculiarities' of sense organ. Aristotle's illusion is a well known example of it. Cross two fingers and, touch a marble, and you seem to feel two marbles. A round ball can be used in place of the marble.

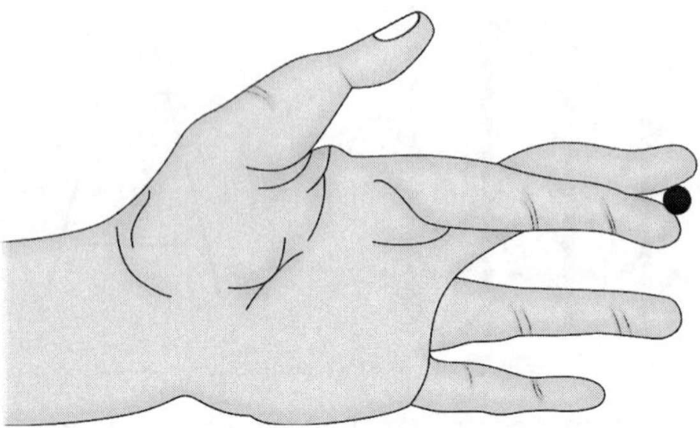

Fig. 3.19: Aristotle's illusion

- **Wrong sign and meaning:** Sometime, misunderstanding of signs lead to illusion. If sign and meaning are not properly understood there could be chances of illusion.
- **Fear:** One is likely to see what one dreads to see. In fear the rope appear in the form of snake and an old and dread tree may be perceived as ghost.
- **Habit and similarity:** Habit and similarity also cause illusion. The best example of this case is *'proofreader's illusion'*, though the professional proofreader is less subject to it. For example, in hurry one can reads 'motivation' as 'motivation'.
- **Similarity:** This is another common cause of illusion. We often mistake one of the twin brothers for the other because of their similarity in physical gesture and body movements.
- **Contrast:** Contrast is again a cause of illusion. A black man perceived more black in presence of white and a tall man perceived more taller in presence of a short-heighted man or vice-versa.
- **Recency:** Illusion may be caused due to recency effect. For example, an experience of earthquake may lead us to perceive a slight tremor of passing a heavy loaded truck as earthquake.
- **Eye movement:** Although many theories exist for this illusion, but there is no certain explanation. One theory based on eye movement. When the arrow point inwards, our gaze rests inside the angles formed by arrows. When they point outwards, our eyes demarcate the entire perspective and out gaze rest outside the angles. The outwards pointing arrows make the figure more open and so the horizontal line appears longer, this phenomena explains in Muller–Lyer illusion.

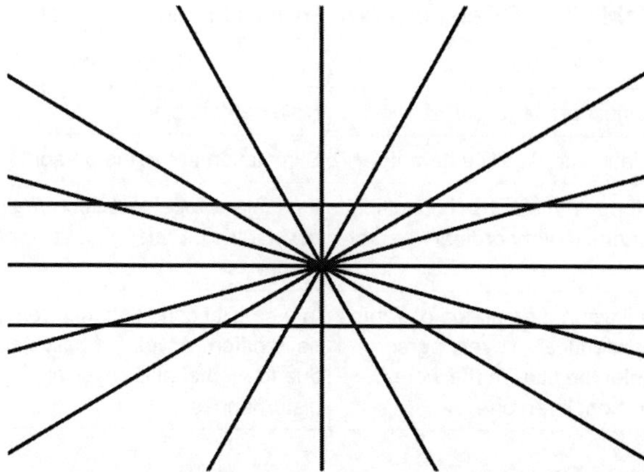

Fig. 3.20: Muller-Lyer illusion

Hallucination

Hallucination is the perceptual experience in the absence of external stimulus. For example, perceiving a coat for ghost hanging on a hook, is illusion but if we see a ghost, even there is no coat, or hook, or anything else, we said to have hallucination. So hallucination is perception of object without is presence.

Types of Hallucination

Following are common hallucinations:

- *Auditory hallucination*: hearing voice that are not present
- *Visual hallucination*: visualization of certain object, subjects, images
- *Gustatory hallucination*: feeling taste of certain things
- *Kinesthetic hallucination*: feeling that something crawling on skin
- *Hypnopompic hallucination*: perception which can occur on falling asleep
- *Hypnogogic hallucination*: perception which can occur on waking up.

Difference between Hallucination and Illusion

Hallucination is dissimilar to illusion. In illusion, external object present, though it wrongly interpreted. When we take a rope for snake, we have an illusion. In illusion, there is a real object is present, though it is presented other than it is. In hallucination, external object/subject perceived without its due presence.

Table 3.3: Difference between illusion and hallucination

Illusion	Hallucination
External object present	No external object
The stimulation is usually external	Stimulation are in the person
Illusion happens in a normal condition. It can happens to very ordinary person	It usually happens in abnormal or psychiatric people, or in case of mental tiredness
In case of illusion, perception of same situation is identical to every person. For example, the stick in the water appears to bent everyone	In a special condition, different people have different types of hallucination due to mental and physical disturbances

Suggested Reading

- Balcetis E, Dunning D. Cognitive dissonance and the perception of natural environments. Psychol Sci. 2007;18(10):917-21.
- Balcetis E, Dunning D. See what you want to see: motivational influences on visual perception. J Pers Soc Psychol. 2006;91(4): 612-25.
- Blakemore SJ, Decety J. From the perception of action to the understanding of intention. Nat Rev Neurosci. 2001;2(8):561-7.
- Bruner JS. On perceptual readiness. Psychol Rev. 1957; 64(2): 123-52.
- Eriksen CW, Yeh YY. Allocation of attention in the visual field. J Exp Psychol Hum Percept Perform. 1985;11(5):583-97.

REVIEW QUESTIONS

SHORT-ESSAY TYPE QUESTIONS

1. Define sensation and discuss the process of sensation.
2. Write the characteristics of sensation.
3. Explain the errors of perception.
4. Discuss various factors that can affect attention.
5. Differentiate hallucination to illusion.
6. Discuss the concept of figure and ground theory.

MULTIPLE CHOICE QUESTIONS

1. It is wrong or misinterpretation of a subject/object?
   a. Illusion b. Hallucination
   c. Delusion d. Disorientation
2. Which of the following is the most common hallucination in psychiatric patient?
   a. Auditory b. Visual
   c. Tactile d. Gustatory
3. Figure and ground theory used while the interpretations of which of the following cognitive function?
   a. Perception b. Sensation
   c. Emotion d. Touch
4. Perception of any stimulus in its absence is called:
   a. Illusion b. Hallucination
   c. Sensation d. Delusion
5. Which of the following belongs to involuntary attention?
   a. Enforced attention b. Implicit attention
   c. Explicit attention d. Selective attention
6. Which of the following term used if an individual focuses on more than one activity?
   a. Selective attention b. Division attention
   c. Habitual attention d. Voluntary attention
7. The figure and ground theory implicate to understand the concept of following:
   a. Sensation b. Perception
   c. Attention d. Hallucination
8. The figure and ground theory was proposed by a group of psychologist known as:
   a. Morris b. Gestalt
   c. Silverman d. Con air
9. The ability to know something in advance of its occurrence or to predict a future event is called:
   a. Clairvoyance b. Rebirth
   c. Precognition d. Telepathy
10. Which of the following is not a nature of attention?
    a. Shifting b. Selective
    c. Imaginary d. Division

11. The psychological school of thought that stressed the whole or complete view of a situation was:
    a. Structuralism
    b. Functionalism
    c. Behaviorism
    d. Gestalt
12. Who established the first psychology lab in the United States?
    a. Stanley Hall
    b. William James
    c. Francis Cecil Sumner
    d. Mary Whiton Calkins

ANSWER KEY

1.	a	2.	a	3.	a	4.	b	5.	a	6.	b	7.	b
8.	b	9.	c	10.	c	11.	d	12.	a				

Learning and its Theories

Chapter 4

INTRODUCTION

Man is a rational being. He has got the power of reasoning. The power of reasoning enables him to learn quickly. Learning play very important role in determining the behavior of an individual. Learning is the basis of success in life. The miracles of the present day civilization are the result of learning. Learning occupies very important place in the field of education. It is through learning that man brings in so many changes in his instincts that it becomes difficult to recognize them.

NATURE OF LEARNING

Meaning of Learning

Learning is said to be equivalent to change, modification, development, improvement and adjustment. It is not limited to school learning, cycling, reading, writing or typing but it is a comprehensive term which leaves permanent effect or impression on individual.

Definition of Learning

'Learning is modification of behavior through experiences'
(Gates)

'Learning involves the acquisition of habits, knowledge and attitude' (Crow and Crow)

'Learning is both acquisition and retention' (Skinner)

'It is a process by which behavior is originated an changed through practice or training' (Garry and Kingsley)

'Any addition to our experience is a kind of learning'
(Woodworth)

In summary, we can say that learning is a fundamental process of life engaging much of our waking hours, affecting all forms of behavior, skills, knowledge, attitude, personality, motivation, fear and mannerism.

It involves:
- Acquisition of new experiences
- Retention of new experiences in the form of impression
- Development of experiences, step-by-step modification of experiences and creation of old and new experiences
- Organization, synthesis and integration of old and new experiences.

Characteristics of Learning

- **Progressive change in behavior:** Learning brings progressive changes in the behavior as the individual reacts to the situation and change himself.
- **Learning is motivated by adjustment:** The individual has to adjust to new environment that push him to learn something.
- **Learning is universal:** All living being on earth involve in learning process.
- **Learning is continuous process:** Learning takes place at any span of life, i.e. childhood, adolescence, adult and old age.
- **Learning is goal directed/purposeful:** When the purpose or goal is more clear, vivid and explicit, the learning become meaningful and affective to learner.
- **Learning is active and creative:** Learning depends on active level of learner. A more active learner learn more quickly than a passive learner.
- **Learning is transferable:** Learning is transferable from one person to another and one place to another. Transfer occurs when there are similarities of content, techniques, ideas, procedures and attitudes.
- **Learning is need based:** Learning largely depend on individual— his needs, interest, problems, attitudes, aspiration and needs of the society.
- **Learning possible at all level:** Learning can be in the form of getting new knowledge (cognition), sharpening of skill/ competencies (psychomotor) and changes in attitude (conative/ affective).
- **Environmental influence change learning:** Children grow in different environment learn in different manner. Environment mould the learner to learn in different manner. For example, children belong to adverse family and socioeconomic condition, i.e. poverty, sometimes shows a wonderful results in learning

outcome, i.e. former Prime Minister Lal Bahadur Sastri is an example of this. Sometimes, children belong to very low socioeconomic condition become fail in education due to non-availability of adequate resources.

- **Learning is a problem solving:** Learning helps the individual to learn new things in order to adjust in the environment. Many personal as well as social problems can be solved with the help of learning.
- **Learning may be right or wrong:** Modification in behavior of an individual depends on types of learning. Improper and inadequate learning leads to maladaptive behavior development in an individual, i.e. terrorist and all.
- **Learning is an individualized process:** Many individual factors may influence successful learning, i.e. memory, thinking, interest, and motivation, etc.
- **Learning is a function of nervous system:** Nervous system and brain play an important role in learning. It is evidenced that complex nervous system helps to learn more efficiently than simple one. It is also understood that damage of particular area of brain may result temporary and permanent loss of the concerned function of the area.
- **Learning is a process not a product:** This can be understood by following steps:
  - **Motives and needs:** First of all motives and needs arise. Motive is a force which impinges or compels the individual to adjust according to situation.
  - **Goal:** If motives or need is there, the goal is set up by the teacher or anyone else.
  - **Adjustment:** Adjustment on the part of learner begins.
  - **Changes:** Changes in the behavior of the individual take place.
  - **Stabilization:** Changes are stabilized in the form of behavior of the individual.

TYPES OF LEARNING

- **Motor learning:** Motor learning take place in the child when his mental capacities are not so developed, i.e. eye-hand coordination, walking, running, jumping, etc. This type of learning takes place through imitation.

- **Perceptual learning:** As the mind grow and mature, the child start getting sensation through different sense organs and gives meaning to them. It means that objects around him are meaningful to him and he perceives them. He learns the name of different object in order to differentiate them.
- **Conceptual learning:** At this stage, the mental capacities are sufficiently developed from its own ideas and concepts. The learning becomes ideational one; power of thinking and judgment is developed. The individual now able to solve problems in his own way.
- **Associate learning:** Conceptual learning is helped by associative learning. New concepts or experience are associated with old or previous concepts and ideas.
- **Appreciational learning:** Appreciational learning is on affective side while conceptual learning is on cognitive side.
- **Attitudinal learning:** The child leans or develops certain attitudes like an attitude of belongingness towards his family and friends and other.

METHODS OF LEARNING

Trial and Error Method

Thorndike (1898), an American Psychologist, given the concept of trial and error theory of learning. He conducted many experiments on cat, dogs, fish and monkeys and concluded that both human being and animals learn many things through trial and error method. It is based on the concept that when we learn begin to learn anything there may be many errors or mistakes in the beginning but as the number of trials goes on increasing, the errors or mistakes goes on decreasing. Thus, we learn from mistakes or experience.

Learning by Insight (Gestalt's View)

Kohler, a German psychologist given this theory. According to this theory, human beings and animals also learn through intelligent observation. He said that all learning take place through insight. Insight means inner sight, seeing deep in to solution of the problem. According to professor Woodworth, 'by insight is meant of good observation, perception of the situation as a whole or perception of those parts of the situation that provide a route to the goals'. In insight learning, whole is more important than the parts. For meaningful organization of objects individual apply different laws.

- **Law of similarity:** That is similarity in form, shape, color, size leads to different meaningful organization of the field.
- **Law of proximity or nearness:** That is things which are near to each other's helps in the organization of the object as whole or in parts.
- **Law of continuity:** That is good continuation helps in organization.
- **Essentials of learning by insight**
  - **Comprehension as a whole:** Learning by insight require full comprehension of the situation as a whole.
  - **Clear goal:** The goal must be clear enough.
  - **Power of generalization:** The learner must possess power of generalization along with those of differentiation.
  - **Suddenness of solution:** Suddenness of solution is the hallmark of learning by insight, i.e. the solution flashes suddenly to the learner.
  - **New form of object:** As a result of insight into the problem or situation, object appear in new form and pattern.
  - **Transfer:** Transfer of learning occur as a result of insight. The principles learnt in one situation are applied to the other situation.
  - **Changes in behavior:** Insight helps to change the behavior.

Learning by Conditioning

The exponent of this was Ivan Pavlov and Watson. According to this theory learning take place by condition. Conditioning implies the attachment or association of original response with the new artificial stimuli. Conditioning is the modification of innate or natural behavior.

Learning by Imitation

Imitation is the oldest method of learning. Both human being and animals learn various things by imitation. Imitation found in all children and adults. Even some and animals imitate. The imitation power of monkey and parrot is well-known. When one sheep goes away, all others follow. In imitation, the learner copies the behavior, habit, manner and way of others. Whenever this copying is observed, it is said that one has learned through imitation.

Characteristics of Learning by Imitation

- **Immediate performance:** The imitator performs the activity at once. He never does it before imitation.
- **No earlier knowledge:** The imitator does not know earlier the activity to be imitated.
- **Exact copying:** In imitation, the learner exactly copies the activities performed before him.

Types of Imitation

- **Simple imitation:** In simple imitation, one aspect of the things or event is imitated. It is used in the acquisition of language by the child.
- **Idealistic imitation:** In this type of imitation, the child imitates things according to the idea that has been put before him.
- **Spontaneous imitation:** The learner imitate thing that are of his interest and liking. For example, when we see a train whistling we also learn to whistle.
- **Dramatic imitation:** The child imitates the things that she hears or sees. For example, she starts playing with the dolls, making them sleep and marrying them.
- **Copying:** In copying, there is complete imitation in all respects. In other words of Prof. Boring, 'copying is an elaborate type of imitation in which no aspect is left out.'

Table 4.1: Comparison of trial and error learning and insightful learning

Trial and error learning	Insight learning
Depends upon efforts of the learner	Depends on insight and intellectual level of learner
Main stress is on physiological efficiency	Main stress on brain functions
Based on sensory-motor to coordination	Based on perception
No transfer of learning	Transfer possible
Available to all	Comparatively confined to those with higher intellectual level
More useful in case of mentally deficient and children	More useful in adults and person having good intellectual level

Observational Learning

Bandura proposed the concept of observational learning. It is learning new behavior through observing the behavior of others. For example, child learning.

Rote Learning

It is learning by repetition. It is also known as parroting. Rote learning avoids understanding the meaning of subject matter and only focuses on memorizing the material so that it can be recalled exactly as it has memorizes.

Informal Learning

This is an unorganized way of learning. In informal learning, learning can take place at anywhere, i.e. home, surrounding and road side.

Formal Learning

Formal learning always takes place at school, college or at some recognized institute.

PROCESS OF LEARNING

Learning is a continuous process. It begins with life and end with life. Learning leads to many changes, adjustment and development in an individual and enable to modify the behavior. It enables an individual to develop necessary new skills and abilities to help in adjustment.

Factors Influencing Learning

Learning is a never ending process and there are a number of factors which may influence the learning process. Broadly, these factors are discussed under following four headings:

1. Factors related to learner
2. Factors related to learning material
3. Factors related to methods of learning
4. Factors related to learning environment.

Factors Related to Learner

The process of learning may vary from individual-to-individual. There are certain individual factors responsible for learning. These are as follows:

- **Age:** It is understood that learning process get slow with advancement of age. The learning capacity is higher in early age and decrease slowly with the advancement of age.
- **Gender:** Gender difference does not cause any difference in their intelligence but may have influence on learning. For example, girls are more proficient in literature, debate and

songs while boys are higher interested in scientific technology and ideological fields.

- **Previous experience:** The present learning depends on the past experiences. It is evidenced that a person with rich past experience enable the individual to learn the material more proficiently. Present learning has consequential impact on future learning.
- **Effect of memorization:** Frequent memorization will help to make the learning lifelong. For example, students who memorize the learning material frequently will able to write and speak more confidently then others.
- **Effect of psychological well-being/mental stability:** Learning and mental stability has direct relations each others. Attention is the key for learning process. A learner should be attentive to learn and understand the phenomena in a whole.
- **Effect of previous learning outcomes:** Frequent failure or negative results gives a feeling of inferiority and helpless in the learner that may decrease learning process. On the other hand successful outcome of learning push the learner to learn the things more robostically. So success and failure have their respective effect on learning process.
- **Interest of learner:** Interest is the most basic necessity for learning. Reading the learning material with interest have higher impact on mind and may result more successful learning.

Factors Related to Learning Material

- **Complexity of subject matter:** Basically, learning should go from simple to complex and should be based on basic principles of teaching-learning process. Following teaching-learning process will helps to make the learning more efficient and interesting.
- **Length of learning material:** It is a well-understood phenomena that learning a short list of words or material will take less time and effort than a long list of lengthy material.
- **Type of subject material:** The meaningful material learned more efficiently than meaningless material.

Factors Related to Methods of Learning

- **Effect of AV aids:** Use of effective, updated and relevant audiovisual aid enable the learning more efficiently.

- **Methods of learning:** Use of different type of teaching methods have different impact on learning outcomes. There are various methods adopted by learner in different age group. For example, imitation is common in kids, drill and practice method is common in students with technological backgrounds and reading and recitation in academic students. Each method of learning has their merits and demerits in teaching-learning process. So, use of appropriate type of method of learning according to age and interest of learner will make learning more efficient and effective.

Factors Related to Learning Environment

There are certain environmental conditions which may influence the learning process, i.e. learning resources—library facilities, use of computer; physical environment—noise level; social environment—social taboos, customs, traditions, socioeconomic condition, social background—urban and rural, etc.

THEORIES OF LEARNING

There are many theories of learning given by psychologists. Some important and relevant theories are explained here:

- **Trial and errors learning theory:** EL Thorndike studied the character of trial and error learning in a number of experiments on cats. He put a cat in a puzzle box with iron bars on the sides. On the floor of the box, a lever was fixed to open the door. A food box was placed outside of the box. The cat was kept hungry for

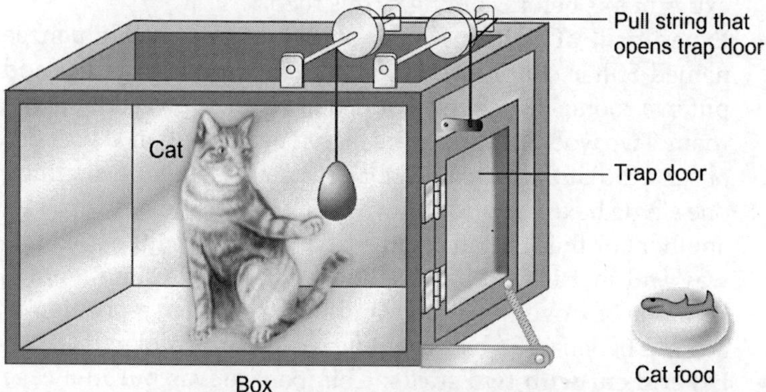

Fig. 4.1: Trial and error learning (cat experiment)

24 hours. The door of the puzzle box was closed. The condition was that cat would only get the food if she learned to press the lever which opened the door. After several unsuccessful attempts, cat finally succeeds to open the door of the box by pressing lever. This same experiments was performed many times and it was seen that at each attempts cat took less time to press the lever and open the door.

- **Dog experiment:** Loyd Morgan put a dog into an iron cage. The door of cage was not clearly visible. The dog made number of attempts before he could open the door.
- **Rat experiment:** McDougall's kept cats in a small box with secret passage. After committing mistakes 165 times, they succeeded in finding out the correct passage.

From the experiment trial and errors, Thorndike formulated following laws:

- **Law of exercise:** According to this law repetition of any response tends to establish or confirm it and if any activity is repeated again and again it is learn effectively.
- **Law of readiness:** According to this law when we are ready to learn, we learn more quickly, effectively and with greater satisfaction than when we are not ready to learn.
- **Law of effort:** According to this law success leads to repetition of a response and the failure to its elimination.
- **Learning of insight theory:** Kohler stressed that learning take place through insight or intellectual level. Insight means seeing deep into the solution of a problem. He conducted many experiments before coming to this theory.
- **Experiment of Sultan:** Kohler experiment on a Chimpanzee named Sultan. In first situation, Sultan was kept hunger and put in a room. He hanged a bunch of bananas on ceiling of the room. Two wooden boxes were placed near to Sultan. It was also observed that Sultan could not get bananas only by standing one single box. The position was such that if one box is put on another box then Sultan could get bananas. So, Sultan tried this way and that way and thought over the whole situation. He kept one box over the others and then he was in a position to achieve bananas. So by insight he solved the problem.
- **Experiment with two sticks:** Chimpanzee was put in a cage and two sticks were kept in the cage. A bunch of bananas were

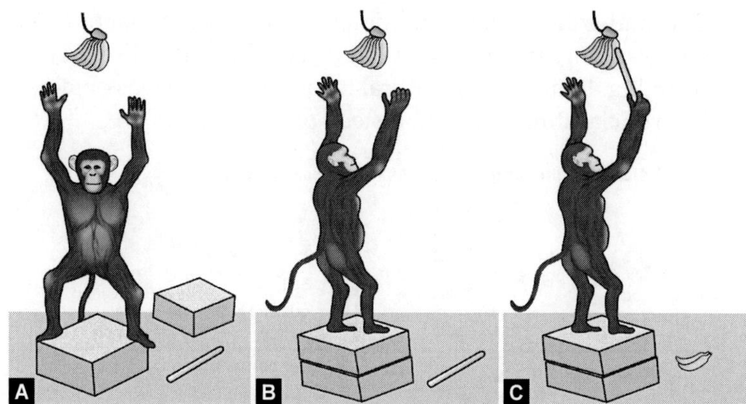

Figs 4.2A to C: Experiment of Sultan

placed outside. The sticks were such if their end could be joined together, they would become one. First, Chimpanzee tried to get bananas with the help of one stick, after many unsuccessful attempt he joins two sticks together and picked up the bananas. So again insight we used to solve the problem.

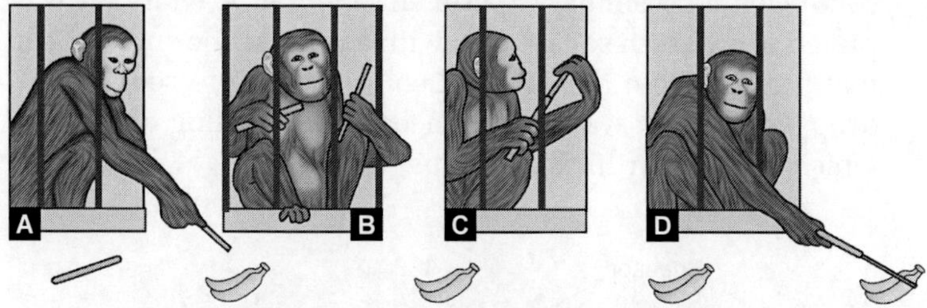

Figs 4.3A to D: Sultan putting two sticks together

- **Classical condition theory of learning:** Classical condition theory was postulated by a Russian Psychologist, Ivan Pavlov and awarded Nobel prize in 1904 for his outstanding achievement in the field of psychology. He said, 'conditioning is nothing but the establishment of connection between a stimulus and a response which have no natural connection between them'.

  Pavlov's dog experiment: Pavlov conducted his experiment on dog. He used to ring the bell before food to the dog. He repeated this activity several times in a day for many days. After some day, under the similar condition, it was observed that only the bell was ring, the food was not placed, but the saliva started secreting. It means that natural response (saliva) was obtained by artificial stimulus (bell) instead of giving food.

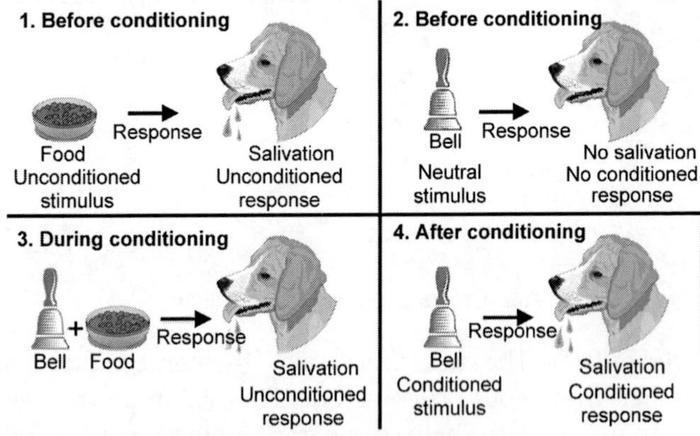

Fig. 4.4: Ivan Pavlov's dog experiment

- **Skinner experiments on rat:** BF Skinner, a Harvard Psychologist, conducted a bit similar experiment on a rat. A white rat was placed in a 12 inch square box, with a lever at one end or a bar that projects from the wall. When the bar is pressed, food is dropped. The rat was conditioned to the pressing of the bar, which act as on artificial stimulus.

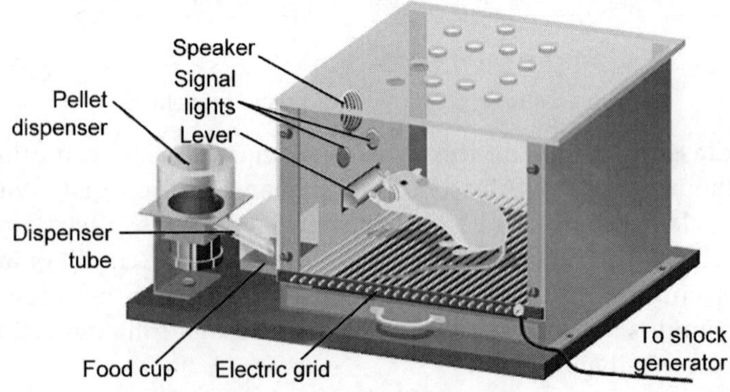

Fig. 4.5: The puzzle box rat experiment

- **Operant conditioning theory:** Operant conditioning theory was given by BF Skinner. This theory was based on a fundamental principle known as reinforcement. Reinforcement means to strengthen the response by rewarding or removal of stimuli. Reinforcement can be positive or negative in nature. He stressed that behavior that is most rewarding is repeated again and again and vice versa. For example, providing chocolate to a child for using toilet when he feels need to use it.

Table 4.2: Classical and operant conditioning compared

Characteristics	Classical conditioning	Operant conditioning
Type of association	Between two stimuli	Between a response and its consequence
State of subject	Passive	Active
Focus of attention	On what precedes response	On what follows response
Type of response typically involved	Involuntary or reflexive response	Voluntary response
Bodily response typically involved	Internal responses: emotional and glandular reactions	External responses: muscular and skeletal movement and verbal responses
Range of responses	Relatively simple	Simple to highly complex
Responses learned	Emotional reactions: fears, likes, dislikes	Goal-oriented responses

TRANSFER OF LEARNING

Transfer is a key concept in education and learning theory because most of formal education aspires to transfer. Process of learning and the transfer of learning are the control to understanding how people develop important competencies. Transfer of learning occur when learning in one context or with one set of material impart or performed in another context or with others. For example, learning to drive a car helps a person to later to learn more quickly to drive a bus or truck. When we talk about the transfer of learning, we are interested in the extent to which learning is transferred from one context to another. Transfer of teaching is often used synonymously with transfer of learning.

Definition

Transfer of learning has been defined in a number of ways. Some important definitions are given here:

'Real transfer happens when people carry over something they learned in one context to a significantly different'.

(Fogarty et al. 1992)

'Transfer is the application of knowledge learned in one setting or for one purpose to another setting and/or purpose.'

(Gange et al. 1993)

Type and Level of Transfer

The levels of transfer often referred to positive and negative one. In addition, in both there are subtle and marked differences in type of transfer. Many of the differences lead to distinction in how transfer is classified depending on the level of complexity of the transfer.

- **Positive versus negative transfer:** When learning in one context improve learning and performance in the another context or situation is called positive transfer. For example, if someone learning to operate new android phone has background knowledge of operating cell phone are likely to benefit in term of time taken to operate the android cell phone. However, negative transfer occurs when previous learning or experience inhibit or interferes with learning or performance in new context. For example, a person with unpleasant schooling experience may avoid classroom situation. It is common for tourists' accustomed to driving on the right hand side of the road to experience difficulty adjusting to driving on the left hand side.
- **Simple versus complex transfer:** Simple transfer happens when no or very little effort is needed to apply what has been learned in our situation to a new situation. In theory class, nursing students are taught how to prepare excel coding sheet for final thesis data entry. Later they need little effort to prepare a master data sheet. However, if some students were engaged in gathering data for research project and thought about the ways in which the master data sheet with data management and analysis, this would be an example of more complex learning.
- **Near and far learning:** Usually, these terms distinguish the closeness of distance between the original learning and the transfer task. For example, learning to shift gears in a truck is an example of near transfer from someone who has already

learned to shift gears in a car. Near transfer has also been seen as the transfer of learning within the school context, or between a school task and very similar task. Far learning is refers to the transfer of learning from school context to nonschool context or home context.

- **Automatic and mindful transfer:** Automatic transfer occurs when an individual respond spontaneously within a transfer situation, which is very similar to the learning situation. For example, learning to read English is one class, results in the learner automatically reading English language in another context. In mindful transfer, the individual need mindful, conscious, deliberate and intellectual efforts to transfer of learning from original context to new context. For example, transfer of demonstration education and training on real clinical setting.

So, we can say that transfer of learning is a pervading concept that is intrinsically linked to the way we lead our lives every day. In fast paced changing society, it is become increasingly important for people to embrace lifelong learning and to be able to transfer what they learned in one context to different context.

Learning and Sickness

Learning and sickness are closely related to each others. As we know that adjustment in day-to-day life needs learning of certain adjustment process. Need of these adjustment process is vary from person-to-person. A sick individual adjustment process will be different than a healthy individual. For example, a person suffering with diabetes mellitus need to learn how to take insulin injection, changes in diet, exercise and other daily routine. Similarly a patient suffering with hypertension also need to learn different adjustment techniques like avoiding salt intake, control on anger, etc.

However, learning certain habits in normal life may predispose to certain disease conditions. For example, learning bad habits of smoking, and alcoholism may predispose many physical and psychological problems, i.e. heart disease, hypertension, addiction, etc. It is also possible for an individual to learn various maladaptive behaviors, i.e. obsessive compulsive behavior, hysterical disorders, and phobia, etc. A person subconsciously may learn certain symptoms, i.e. feeling of weakness, abdominal pain, and mental exhaustion to win sympathy of others and get relief from hectic daily schedule. Learning such maladaptive behavior further complicates the life and has negative impact on personality.

Implications of Learning in Nursing

Nursing is another name of serving humanity. Nursing deals with care and treatment of diseased one. A patient may seek medical advice for many reasons, i.e. physical problem, psychological problem, injury, and behavioral disorders. In this view, a nurse should be well-trained in all the methods, theories and techniques of learning to provide a comprehensive care to their patient. Adequate knowledge of different learning methods and theories will help a nurse to learn new things. For example, nursing procedures based on different theories and methods of learning, giving injection based on conditioning theory of learning and doing demonstration based on trial and error method of learning.

Learning various principles and laws of learning will help a nurse to motivate the patient to help in recovery. Rewarding behavior accordingly during sickness have positive outcome on recovery and discharge. For example, showing excessive sympathy may help the patient to assume a sick role for very long time and delay the recovery while motivating same patient for healthy daily habits, i.e. daily exercise, quitting smoking and abstinence alcohol, may help in speedy recovery.

Suggested Reading

- Anthikad J. Psychology for Graduate Nurses, 4th edn. New Delhi: Jaypee Brothers Medical Publishers (P) Ltd, 2008.
- Bower GH, Hilgard ER. Theories of Learning (5th Edn). NJ: Prentice Hall, 1981.
- Engle RW, Cantor J, Carullo JJ. Individual differences in working memory and comprehension: a test of four hypotheses. J Exp Psychol Learn Mem Cogn. 1992;18(5):972-92.
- Hilgard ER. Introduction to Psychology. New York: Harcourt, Brace and World, 1977.
- Kohler W. Gestalt Psychology. New York: Liveright, 1947.
- Kohler W. Mentality of Apes. London: Routledge & Kegan. 1925; p 128.
- Lamberth J. Foundations of Psychology. New York: Harper and Row Publishers, 1996.

- Morgan CT, King RA, Weisz JR, Schopler J. Introduction to Psychology, 7th edn. New Delhi: Tata McGraw Hill Publishing Company Ltd, 2007.
- Morris, C. Psychology: An Introduction. New Jersey: Prentice Hall, 1980.
- Plotnik R. Introduction to Psychology, 5th edn. USA: Wadsworth Publishing Company, 1998.

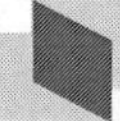

REVIEW QUESTIONS

SHORT-ESSAY TYPE QUESTIONS

1. Define learning. Discuss characteristics of learning.
2. Discuss the factors affecting learning.
3. Discuss types of learning.
4. Explain methods of learning.
5. Explain classical conditioning theory of learning given by Ivan Pavlov.
6. Discuss trial and error theory of learning.

MULTIPLE CHOICE QUESTIONS

1. Thorndike (1898) proposed the concept of following learning theory:
   a. Imitation
   b. Trial and error
   c. Learning of insight
   d. Conditioning theory of learning
2. It is a type of learning in which new concepts or experience are associated with old or previous concepts and ideas:
   a. Rote learning b. Conceptual learning
   c. Associate learning d. Remote learning
3. 'Classical conditioning' theory of learning was proposed by:
   a. Thorndike b. Watson
   c. Ernold d. Ivan Pavlov
4. The process of modifying an individual behavior through experience is called:

a. Transfer of learning
b. Extinction
c. Teaching
d. Learning

5. The reinforcement condition that increase the probability of occurrence of a particular behavior is called:
   a. Negative reinforcement
   b. Positive reinforcement
   c. Punishment
   d. Neutral reinforcement
6. Which of the following psychologist not associated with behaviorism?
   a. JB Watson
   b. Ivan Pavlov
   c. BF Skinner
   d. Bandura
7. The mental image that represents a generalized idea about something is called:
   a. Problems
   b. Thinking
   c. Concept
   d. Perception
8. This learning avoid understanding the meaning of subject matter and only focuses on memorizing the material:
   a. Informal learning
   b. Rote learning
   c. Conditioning learning
   d. Observational learning
9. Which type of learning can be seen in children?
   a. Imitation
   b. Rote learning
   c. Observational learning
   d. Conditioning
10. Once the mental capacities are sufficiently developed and the learning becomes ideational one is known which type of learning?
    a. Motor learning
    b. Perceptual learning
    c. Conceptual learning
    d. Associate learning

ANSWER KEY

1.	b	2.	c	3.	d	4.	d	5.	b	6.	d	7.	c
8.	b	9.	a	10.	b								

Memory and Forgetting

Chapter 5

MEMORY

Man is said to be crown of creation. He has teen endowed with the higher power of memory. It is memory which helps him to take part in imagination, thinking and reasoning. The success, efficiency and durability of learning to a great extent depend on memory. In fact the cause of his superiority over other living organisms, i.e. animals is his highly developed memory. Memory plays a very important role in everyday life. If the man had no memory power, his life too, would have been like that of a lower animal. In that situation he could not learned anything. So it is difficult to imagine the condition of human being without memory power.

NATURE OF MEMORY

Meaning and Definition

Memory is the reproduction of past personal experience in the same order and form. Through memory, past experiences become a living force in the manner in which they were previously experienced. It is the force which helps to bring past experiences to a state of consciousness in the shape of images and ideas.

Definition

'To memories is to remember or reproduce a thing after learning.' (Woodworth)

'It is the ability of the organism to store information from earlier learning process and experience, retention, and reproduction to that information in answer to specific stimuli.' (Eysenk)

'Memories is to show in present responses signs of earlier learned responses'. (Hilgard and Atkinson)

So, on the basis of above definitions we can conclude that memory is a complex cognitive process involving learning retention and recognition. Memory helps to modify the behavior on the basis of experiences gained for something in the memory.

Characteristics of Memory

- Memory is the reproduction of past experience in the same order and form
- Memory originate from learning
- Memory involves learning, retention, recall and recognition
- Memory helps an individual in better living and adjustment
- Memory is constructive
- Memory goes on in the mind of man.

Characteristics of Good Memory

A good memory characterized by following:

- **Accurate and quick:** Learned well is remembered well. One who can learn material accurately and quickly is credited with a good memory. Good memory economy labor and time.
- **Accurate and durable attention:** A good memory concerned with retention of learned material for a long time. The more accurate and durable memory is believed to be good memory.
- **Accurate and quick recall:** Accurate and quick recall deals with good and sharp memory. If it is possible to learn the material accurately and quickly, retain it accurately and quickly; able recall the matter quickly and accurately, then it is called good memory.
- **Accurate and quick recall:** A student should possess the ability to recognize quickly and accurately.
- **Purposefulness:** A person with good memory will remember things that are relevant to the occasion. He is able to recall the relevant material.

TYPES OF MEMORY

Broadly, memory classified in following types:

- **Short-term memory (STM):** In STM, the memory is held for very brief periods of time. It may range from few seconds to few minutes. In this memory, the learnt material is retained in the brain in the form of circular neural connection which can be broken easily by extrinsic factors. The material is retained as long on the bioelectric channel keep as circulating in the neural circuit. As the neural circuit is broken, material is forgotten. For example, dialing a telephone number and afterwards forgetting. For example, a person can easily recall what he had in breakfast, what he had in dinner yesterday, etc.

- **Long-term memory (LTM):** In LTM, the memory is held more or less permanently. It is unlimited in capacity. The material is retained for many minutes, hours, days, months, years and decades. LTM depends on the law of association. The more the learned material is associated with other ideas in the mind, the greater is the permanency. For example, a person can easily recall his date of birth, date of anniversary, etc.
- **Personal and impersonal memory:** Personal memory concerned with recalling of personal events and experiences while impersonal memory concerned with recalling of events, images or things concerned to impersonal memory.
- **Rote and logical memory:** In rote memory, things are learned without understanding the meaning of things or objects. It is also known as *parroting.* In the logical memory, the things are learned on the basis of logical memory, insight and understanding. Rote memory is for short span of time while logical memory is lifelong.
- **Active and passive memory:** Active memory based on efforts and attempts used to recall the learned material while in passive memory, person do not use any effort to recall the learned material.
- **Physiological and psychological memory:** Sometimes, it is possible to do certain task without help of paying attention like typing, driving and cycling, etc. is called physiological memory. If a particular thing is recalled quickly in same order in which it was learned, it is called psychological memory. This is the best memory evidenced by psychologist.

PROCESS OF MEMORY

To explain the process of memory, researchers put forth many models and theories. The most accepted models of memory process are:

1. Information processing model
2. Neurocognitive theory.

Information Processing Model (IPM)

This model focuses on the way the information is processed or handled through encoding, storage and retrieval stages of memory. It assumes that how long a memory will be remembered depends on the stage of memory in which it is stored. According to information processing model, data are encoded in brain as like computer can understand and use. The computer stores that information on a memory disk and then the data are retrieved out of storage as needed. This model primarily proposed three stages of memory systems as: i. sensory memory, ii. short-term memory, and iii. long-term memory.

Steps of Information Processing

- **Encoding:** Encoding refer to retention of material in the brain. Encoding can be in the form of visual, acoustic and semantic. In visual encoding, the learning material retained in the form of visual images, i.e. pictures, personality makeup, face, height and weight. Acoustic encoding refers to retention of the material in the form of sound, i.e. voice, sound, tune, rhythm, etc. Semantic encoding understands the meaning of the thing and retain it, i.e. concept of balanced diet, concept of malnutrition, etc. So, with this discussion it is clear that STM memory retain the material in the form of visual and sound and LTM retain the memory in the form of meaning and very less in the form of sound and images.

Breaking 'memory' into a series of steps in a process

Three steps, or stages
1. You put stuff in. (encoding)
2. It stays there. (storage)
3. You get it out. (retrieval)

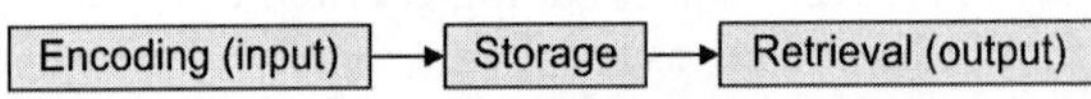

Fig. 5.1: Information processing system

- **Storage:** Storage is the heart of memory processing. The storage capacity of long-term and short-term memory is vary. Normally, sensory or short-term memory store information in seven letter or digits or *chunks*. A chunk is a meaningful unit of information built from smaller piece of information and *chunking* is the process of creating a new chunk. Thus, chunk is a collection of materials that have strong association with one another and is considered as one unit. For example, the mobile number 9876974501 may be retained in the form of 987-697-4501 or 98769-74501. *Mnemonics* is another way of organization of material. For example, name of essential amino acid is very difficult to remember, but help of mnemonics make it easy to store and recall. For example, phenylalanine, valine, threonine, tryptophan, methionine, leucine, isoleucine, histidine and lysine, these can be remembered easily by mnemonics PVT TIM HALL.

The duration of retention of learning material depend on rehearsal or on exercising the material. Rehearsal may be *mechanical* or *elaborative.* Mechanical rehearsal deals with repeating material again and again without understanding the meaning of material, i.e. rote memory. Elaborative rehearsal refers to understanding the meaning of material and retaining it. Elaborative rehearsal is more effective for long-term storage.

Table 5.1: Memory stores

Features	Short-term memory	Working memory	Long-term memory
Encoding	Copy	Phonemic	Semantic
Capacity	Limited	7±2 chunks	Very large
Duration	0.25 sec	20 sec	Months to year

- **Retrieval:** To recall the material from short-term memory, a person do not to take much effort. It is readymade material in conscious mind and its take minimum time. Recall of learning material from long-term memory will considerably take much more time. It is well-understood that storage of learning material takes in the form of hierarchy. So, retrieval will be in same order. The material which is recently learned will be recalled more easily than the past or old learned material. Sometime, a person not able to recall the material learned before a long time ago. This failure to recall is known as *forgetting.*

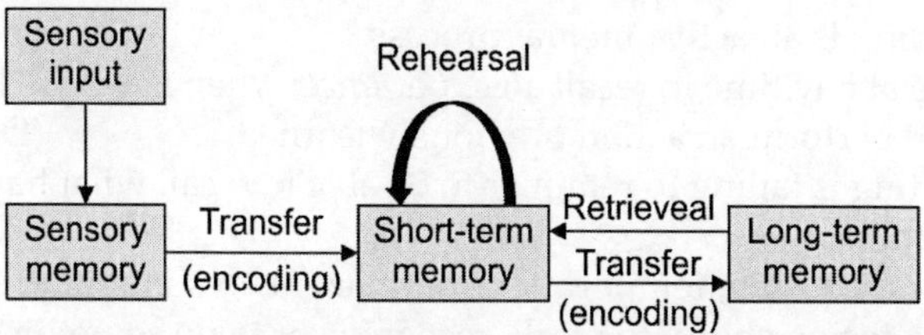

Fig. 5.2: Process of memory

The Neurocognitive Theory

This model focuses on involvement of brain in whole memory process. Memory process involves the plotting of functions on the different parts of the brain. In brain, three sites seem to be directly involved in memory system. These sites are the *cortex* of the brain thought to be involved in higher-order cognition such as thinking, problem solving and remembering; the *cerebellum* at the base of the brain involved in the regulation of motor functions and motor memory; and the *hippocampus* is believed to process new information and route it to parts of the cortex for permanent storage.

FORGETTING

Memory as well as forgetting is important in life. If forgetting does not take place, the life will be burdened with unpleasant experience and become miserable. Fast forgetting is also hinder day-to-day life. So, the amount and speed of forgetting should be reasonable for survival.

Meaning of Forgetting

By forgetting we mean the failure to recall and recognize an idea. It is opposite of memorizing. It is essential for survival as memory.

Ebbinghaus conducted many experiments on forgetting and concluded that forgetting is very rapid immediately after the memorization and then it decrease slightly. He gave the following results of his experiments:

After 20 minutes = 72% retained
After 1 hour = 44% retained
After 6 days = 36% retained
After 1 month = 21% retained

Definition

'Forgetting is an active mental process.' (Woodworth)

'Failure at any time to recall an experience; when attempted to do so, or to perform an action previously learned.' (Drever)

'Forgetting is failing to retain or to be able to recall what has been acquired.' (Munn)

'Loss or the losing, temporary or permanent, of something earlier learned, losing ability to recall, recognize or to do something.' (English and English)

Types of Forgetting

- **Normal or natural forgetting:** It is not possible to retain each and every incident and we forget each day something. This is due to disuse of material. The memory traces become fainter and fainter with less possible of time and the bonds between the nerves which are formed as a result of memorization become also weaker and weaker.
- **Active forgetting:** The person knowingly do not want to recall some unpleasant or unrelated experiences, i.e. bad memories, worst outcome, etc.
- **Passive forgetting:** Forgetting is a natural process and comes automatically. In passive forgetting, the person forgets the things without making any effort.
- **Abnormal forgetting:** Abnormal forgetting is bit similar to active forgetting. The concept of abnormal forgetting was given by Sigmund Freud. According to his version, forgetting is due to conscious repression by the subject. There are certain experiences and memories which are unpleasant and painful to us and we do not want to retain them in mind for long time. The result is that they are deliberately repressed in the unconscious mind.
- **Theories of forgetting:** Exact process of forgetting is still unclear. Many psychologists proposed different views about forgetting process and some of their views are discussed here. These are:
  - **Memory trace decay theory:** This is a very old theory explain process of forgetting. According to this theory, as the time pass the neural bond of memory become weak and weak and fade away that leads to forgetting. This causes forgetting.
  - **Interference theory:** According to this theory, forgetting results due to interference between storing of new and existing old memories. Interference may be retroactive and proactive interference. In retroactive interference, information currently being learned interferes with information already present in memory. For example, learning an advanced android cell phone program cause to forget the already learned old cell phone program. In proactive interference, the previously learned information present in long-term memory interferes with information which we are learning at present. For example, suppose you

learned how to operate one TV, now you buy a new one, which requires different steps to operate. If you now make mistakes by trying to operate the new TV in the same way as you did the old, this constitutes proactive interference.

IMPROVEMENT OF MEMORY OR MEMORY TRAINING

Improvement or training of memory is a controversial issue so far. Modern psychologists believe that memory is gifted power. Hence, it is not possible to improve or train it by practice. William James said that retention is a psychological gift which depends on physiological structure of the individual. Modern psychologist believe that memory cannot be improved but they admit that sing certain methods will help in better memorization and recall.

- **Making association:** Making association is conductive to memorization. It is always good to follow the principle of association in learning and memorization. For example, VIBGYOR can be very useful in memorizing the colors of spectrum.
- **Linking current knowledge with old:** New knowledge should be linked with the previous learned knowledge and experience to make it remember and delay forgetting. It will helps to retain the material in mind and enable recall quickly.
- **Persistent revision:** *'Practice makes a man perfect'* is an ancient proverb to justify that persistent revision makes the memory sharp and quick for particular material. Repetition of learning material timely will makes the memory quick and accurate.
- **Learning by doing:** Learning by doing facilitate memory and easy recall. An old Chinese proverb justifies this;

  If I hear....... I forget
  If I see........ I remember
  If I do...... I understand.

  This applies to teaching somebody something. It means that if you simply talk about something to a person, it is very likely that he will forget what was said. If you tell them and show them, they will more likely remember what was taught. If you involve them in a 'hands on activity/manner', they will fully understand and able to recall it as it is.
- **Whole learning:** Learning the incident or things as a whole will give you more permanent and accurate memory for that material. This will helps to make association between different

parts of the lesson. For example, reading a disease condition step-by-step, i.e. introduction, etiology, signs/symptoms, investigation and management.

- **Introducing rest in between:** Giving rest between learning will facilitates quicker and long-lasting memory. Rest improves fatigues, monotony and refreshes of mind.
- **Use of proper grouping:** Grouping facilitate remembering and memorization. For example, memorization of a telephone or mobile number in chunks rather than whole, i.e. it is easy to remember the mobile number in two or three kind of groupings, i.e. 98769-74501 or 987-679-4501.
- **Use of reinforcement:** A designed kind of reinforcement (positive or negative) will facilitates learning as well memory. For example, fear of getting fail in exams will improve the learning and memorization during exams days.
- **Motivation:** Motivation creates interest in learner. It facilitates capturing, attention, learning and memorization.
- **Meaningful learning:** Intelligent and meaningful learning is more conducive to memorization. Hence, a teacher should focus on lesson rather than irrelevant or trivial discussion in class.
- **Use of rhyme:** It has been seen that children remember effectively the multiplication tables and poem in the sing song fashion.

FACTORS CAUSING FORGETTING

- **Age and forgetting:** Advancement in age associated with decrease learning, retention and more forgetfulness.
- **Meaningfulness of material:** A more meaningful material is more quickly and easily learned and memorized than nonsense, irrelevant and disconnected material.
- **Passage of time:** Time is an important factor responsible for forgetting. As Ebbinghaus found in his experiments that after 20 minutes 72% learned material retained, after 1 hour 44%, after 6 days 36% and after 1 month only 21% material is retained. So, as the time pass memory links goes weak and breaks and we gradually forget the material.
- **Lack of revision:** Lack of revision of learned material leads to forgetting. So, things are forgotten due to lack of practice or repetition and revision.

- **Over learning:** Over learning without proper spacing strain our nerves and is easily forgotten.
- **Loss of interest:** Loss of interest in any activity will no longer helps to retain the learned materials.

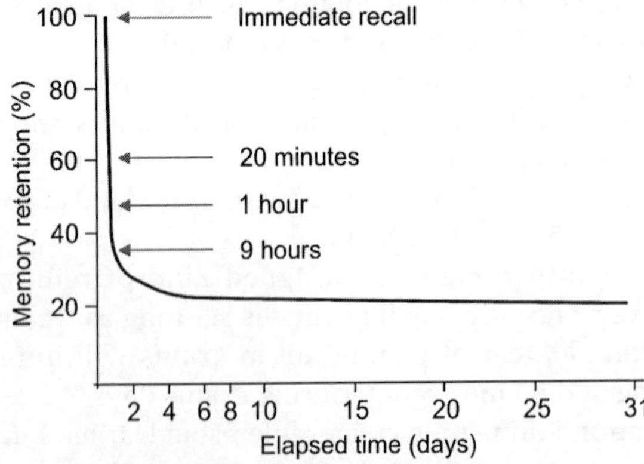

Fig. 5.3: The forgetting curve

The 'forgetting curve' was developed by Hermann Ebbinghaus in 1885. Ebbinghaus memorized a series of nonsense syllables and then tested his memory of them at various periods ranging from 20 minutes to 31 days. This simple but landmark reserch project was the first to demonstrate that there is an exponential loss of memory unless information is reinforced.

Source: Stahl SM, Davis RL, Kim DH, et al. Play it Again: The Master Psychopharmacology Program as an Example of Interval Learning in Bite-Sized Portions. CNS Spectr. 2010;15(8):491-504.

- **Pathological forgetting:** Psychoanalytical theory emphasized that forgetting take place due to deliberate repression of certain undesirable and painful experiences.
- **Degree of learning:** The task learned below the required limit will be retained for a shorter time spans compared to the task which learnt above or at the required limit.
- **Emotional factors:** Certain emotional factors like pain, anger, are likely associated to forget the learned material.
- **Natures of task:** Meaningful, pleasant and easy task are easily recalled than a unpleasant, complex and boredom task.
- **Fatigue:** Fatigue and forgetfulness related to each other. Fatigue leads to accumulation of poisonous substances and affects the memory.
- **Retroactive inhibition:** Retroactive inhibition play an important role in forgetting. Retroactive inhibition is the interference with

retention of learning material in the brain. The interference of old material with the new one is called proactive inhibition. They are many situations which may affect proactive inhibition;

- **Similarity of task or material:** The more the similarity between old and new task or material, the more the retroactive inhibition; hence lesser retention of the original material and more forgetting.
- **Degree of learning:** Over learning of a task tend to interfere in retaining of material, hence forgetting is impaired.
- **Amount of learnt material:** Increase amount of learning material may interfere in the existing learned material in mind.
- **Mental set:** A strong and desire mental set and psychological preparedness facilitates learning.
- **Simultaneous performance:** The amount of interference is maximized when two task are learned simultaneously.

MEMORY AND SICKNESS

Sickness has direct relation with cognitive functions of human being. Sickness can have direct and indirect effect on the memory process. Sometime patient find difficult to learned and retain new things and on some other time it is difficult for same patient to recall and memorizing the things. For example, in case of amnesia it is very difficult for a person to recall the things very timely. Amnesia can be of following types:

- **Localized amnesia:** In some cases, memory loss is related to some particular event or incident. For example, a person suffering with localized amnesia not able to recall particular event only, i.e. memory related to particular festival, marriage party, etc.
- **Generalized amnesia:** In this amnesia, a person not able to recall anything of his past. He lost all his memories. Generalized amnesia could be due to severe psychotic disorders, long-term coma, or may be due to brain damage.
- **Retrograde amnesia:** In retrograde amnesia, the memory loss is restricted before a particular incident. For example, a person not able to recall anything of his schooling.
- **Anterograde amnesia:** In anterograde amnesia, the memory loss is limited to the experiences happened just after accident. For example, a person not able to recall anything after his 10th birthday dates.

There could be many other organic psychiatric disorders which may have direct impact on memory functioning, i.e. Korsakoff syndrome and transient global amnesia. *Korsakoff syndrome* is a profound amnesia, which is normally caused by chronic alcoholism. Those with this disorder usually suffer from some retrograde amnesia as well, but their primary deficit is the inability to store any new information in long-term memory. *Transient global amnesia* is characterized by temporary variation in memory recalling due to migraine and transient ischemic attack.

MEMORY AND NURSING

Memory is essential cognitive aspect for a nurse working in hospital setting. She has to remember many things while providing care to patients, i.e. name of drug, dose, side effect, emergency treatment, many medical and technical terms, duty hours and many more orders to carry out comprehensive care.

It is usual in a hospital to keep on changing the patient and their related information, i.e. name, age, diagnosis, treatment, investigation report and drugs orders. So, a nurse should have intact memory to keep all the information remember and provide consistent care. Sometime poor memory leads hazardous consequences in clinical area. In that view, performance with intact memory will help to overcome many bad consequences and save life of patient and nurse as well. In case of poor memory, a nurse can use following measures to avoid negligence and bad consequences:

- It is better to keep a small diary to write down information to cross check whenever she feels need
- She should cross check all the order before proceeding to it
- In case of some doubt use help of concerned authority
- Use standard abbreviation and do not use own created abbreviation to avoid any mistake.

So, memory is an essential and important cognitive aspect for nursing personnel.

Suggested Reading

- Bhatia BD, Craig M. Elements of Psychology and Mental Health, 1st edn. Hyderabad, Orient Longman, 2006.
- Miller GA. The magical number seven plus or minus two: some limits on our capacity for processing information. Psychol Rev. 1956;63(2):81-97.

- Morgan CT, King RA, Weisz JR, et al. Introduction to Psychology, 7th edn. New Delhi: Tata McGraw Hill Publishing Company Ltd, 2007.
- Rohrer D, Wixted JT, Salmon DP, et al. Retrieval from Semantic Memory and Its Implications in Alzheimer's Disease. Journal of Experimental Psychology: Learning, Memory, and Cognition, 1995;21:1127-39.

REVIEW QUESTIONS

SHORT-ESSAY TYPE QUESTIONS

1. Define memory and factors influencing memory process.
2. Define forgetting and explain theory of forgetting.
3. Discuss types of memory.
4. Discuss disorder related to memory.

MULTIPLE CHOICE QUESTIONS

1. Which of the following method of memory called parroting?
   a. Mnemonic
   b. Whole versus part method
   c. Space versus unspace method
   d. Recitation method
2. The past learning method interfere in the recall of recent learning material is called:
   a. Proactive inhibition b. Retroactive inhibition
   c. Repression d. Trace decay
3. The memory theory of forgetting related to passage of time is given by:
   a. Ebbinghaus b. Woodworth
   c. Drever d. Munn
4. Which of the following is called temporary memory?
   a. Short-term memory b. Long-term memory
   c. Semantic memory d. Episodic memory
5. It is a type of amnesia that involve lapse of memory related to past events:

a. Anterograde amnesia
b. Retrograde amnesia
c. Transient amnesia
d. Localized amnesia

6. In which of following types of encoding the retention of the material takes place in the form of sound, tune and rhythm?
   a. Acoustic
   b. Visual
   c. Spatial
   d. Semantic
7. This memory is held for very brief periods of time. It may range from few seconds to few minutes. It is called:
   a. Short-term memory
   b. Long-term memory
   c. Semantic memory
   d. Episodic memory
8. It is a meaningful unit of information built from smaller piece of information and collection of materials that have strong association with one another. It is called:
   a. Chunks
   b. Mnemonics
   c. Block
   d. Cortex

ANSWER KEY

1.	d	2.	b	3.	a	4.	a	5.	b	6.	a	7.	a
8.	a												

Chapter 6

Thinking

INTRODUCTION

Thinking is the most basic set of cognitive processes of human mind. During most of our waking hours and even when we are in sleep and dreaming, we are thinking; we can say that it is hard not to think. What do we do when we think? Loosely speaking, we might say that we mentally or cognitively process information. More formally, we can say that thinking consists of cognitive re-arrangement or manipulation of both information from the environment and the symbols stored in the long-term memory. From another point of view, thinking is the form of information process that goes on during the period between a stimulus vents and the response to it.

DEFINITION

'Thinking is a behavior which often implicit and hidden in which symbols (images, ideas and concepts) are ordinarily employed.' (Garrett, 1968)

'Thinking is a problem-solving process in which we use ideas or symbols in place of overt activity'. (Glimer, 1970)

'Thinking is an implicit problem-solving behavior.' (Mohsin)

THE PROCESS OF THINKING

Thinking is increasingly complex and difficult concept to discuss and explain in psychology. Thinking can be grounded as a intermediate stage between a stimulus and a response. Developmentally, a child thinking is much more simpler and progress to complex thinking as child grow up. Technically speaking, thinking helps us to remember or reactivate a previously made symbolic connection between learning attentively and solving the problem.

On the other hand, thinking is a mental process of solving problems. It includes an array of thoughts continue to come one after another and this internal process continue till thoughts are expressed in the form of action or language.

TYPES OF THINKING

There are many different kind of thinking possible. Some of the common kinds of thinking are discussed here:

- **Positive thinking:** This kind of thinking concerned with positive thoughts and ideas and positive life outcomes. Positive thinking has direct relation with good mental health.
- **Negative thinking:** Negative thinking is opposite to positive thinking where a person is always dominant with negative thoughts and ideas and never thinking for positive aspects of life. Long-term negative thinking is a poor indicator of good mental health.
- **Critical thinking:** Critical thinking involves a combination of positive and negative thoughts for someone or something. A person with critical thinking evaluates the person or things with both aspects and reaches in conclusion. Critical thinking needs lot of experience in life.
- **Convergent thinking:** In this kind of thinking, an individual think for a problem on different point or angle and try to converge those ideas into one common ground in order to find a solution for the problem. This is particularly true when the problem do not have a single solution.
- **Divergent thinking:** This kind of thinking is opposite to convergent thinking. In this thinking a person start with a common point and move outwards in a verity of perspective. On the other hand we can say that a person start with a common goal and move to very specific.
- **Inductive thinking:** In this type of thinking the process start from part to whole or specific to general to find solution to a problem.
- **Deductive thinking:** This type of thinking starts from many specific alternatives or solution and end with combination of these alternatives to make a common solution to the given problem.

LEVEL OF THINKING

Level of thinking depends on complexity of given problem. Different problem involve different level of thinking. Bloom's taxonomy described following level of thinking.

- **Level I—Knowledge:** This level concerned with recalling of previous learned material.
- **Level II—Comprehension:** This refers to understanding facts by comparison, translation, and interpretation of main ideas.
- **Level III—Application:** This involves application of knowledge to solve a problem.
- **Level IV—Analysis:** This level of thinking examine the problem by breaking down its in parts and identifying and understanding it.
- **Level V—Synthesis:** This is opposite to analysis. This involves combining the parts of problem together and proposing alternative solution.
- **Level VI—Evaluation:** This is the highest level of thinking. This process includes making judgment about information validity of ideas on a set of criteria.

BUILDING BLOCKS OF THOUGHT/THINKING

When you think about a problem, you may have a complex statement about, i.e. image of phenomenon, voice, language and other concepts related to phenomena. Thinking process involves all these elements of phenomena together to reach on some conclusions. These basic elements are called as building block of thought or elements of thought. Some of the important elements of thought are discussed here:

- **Concepts:** Concepts are mental image of a phenomena or object which helps to differentiate that thing to the other things. For example, when you think about a lion—you may think dangerous, long jump, sharp teeth, wild animal and king of jungle, etc. These concepts helps you to differentiate the perception of lion from other animal of jungle.
- **Image:** Image is a mind set, a picture or experience of life. An image is a mental representation of some sensory experience. Like everyone remember Hitler as autocratic and most ruler person so far. This autocratic and ruler is an image of Hitler in mind of all.
- **Language:** Human language is a flexible system to communicate our ideas to others. It is well-understood fact that when we hear, read or listen something or someone, we start thinking about it. For example, when we involve in some conversation, we start thinking simultaneously, so language broaden the thinking process.

FACTORS INFLUENCING THINKING PROCESS

Every individual is not a born thinker. He has to learn and adapt many ways of thinking to survive. There are many factors which may influence thinking process. Some of the factors are explained here:

- **Interest and attention:** Interest and attention are basic pre-requisite for thinking. Attention is difficult in case of lack of interest. So, without attention and interest thinking is not possible.
- **Motivation:** Motivation is an inner desire to learn or to look forwards. Motivation enables a person to maintain enthusiasm and give energy to think for findings solution.
- **Emotion:** Emotion influence thinking. Even thinking in strong emotion will be extremely one-sided or biased. Sometimes, faint emotion may speed up the thinking process. So, controlled emotion helps to think rationally.
- **Superstition and prejudice:** Superstition and prejudice influence thinking process and had a detrimental effect on human brain. Superstitions are unreasonable belief about something that would not let the person to think outside of the boundaries of superstition. On the other hand prejudices are some preconceived idea about something or someone. These prejudices may also hinder the normal thinking process.
- **Flexible time limit:** A normal thinking process should not limited to a rigid time frame. A relaxed mind person can think more logically. So, having a flexible time schedule for thinking enable the individual to think more appropriately.
- **Level of intelligence:** This is well-known fact that a person with high intelligence level can think more properly than a feeble minded person.
- **Knowledge and past experiences:** An adequate storage of knowledge and past experiences speed up the normal thinking process.
- **Physical problems and fatigue:** 'A sound mind lives in a sound body' is a well-known ancient proverb value the relationship of body and mind or thinking process. So, for normal and reasonable thinking, a sound mind and physical fitness are basic necessity.

RELATIONSHIP WITH LANGUAGE AND COMMUNICATION

Communication is an essential part of daily life and it is evidenced that since morning to evening around 80% time we spend in communication. Language is a means of communication to convey ideas, expression, needs, feelings, demands and desires. Moreover, verbal communication use language and nonverbal communication has very narrow scope of language. Nonverbal communication use symbols, expression, body language, images, and signs to convey the meaning of communication. Language encompasses every means of communication, i.e. reading, writing, and speaking, etc. In other words we can say that language is a tool to convey or communicate the ideas, gestures, feelings, and needs by speaking. Thus, it can be said that speech is a special form of language and it is depend on concerned language and accent. But language is more effective and stronger than speech as speech could be mumbled or confused one that does not convey any meaning. So, learning and speaking a language properly will be effective way of communicating the needs.

Thinking and language are related to each other. Thinking is the initial requisite to speak something by using appropriate language. Even thinking stimulates a person to speak out. You might have observed something in your daily life that while working on some project, some people start speaking suddenly. In case of lack of language, thinking is just like self talk or brain talk. So, we can say that capability of thinking is related to power of language. It is difficult to think in the absence of language.

THINKING AND SICKNESS

Sickness has direct impact on physiological as well psychological functioning of human being. In case of severe sickness, especially of mental disorders, the thinking is grossly disturbed. For example, a severe psychotic disorder, i.e. schizophrenia, have direct impact on thinking. It leads to disorientation, confusion, paranoid thinking, and delusional types of thinking. Sometimes, some of neurotic disorders also predispose changes in thinking process like obsessive disorder, where a person has irritative, irrational and repetitive thoughts about a particular person or thing. The person preoccupied with the thoughts of a particular thing. This kind of thinking process leads to disturbance in personal, occupation and social life.

Severe depression may also have direct impact on thinking process. A patient with severe depression may have thought of suicide or other negative thoughts like hopelessness, helplessness and no meaning of life. This kind of deviant thinking process will never let the person to come to their normal stage.

There are many other psychiatric disorders that have direct relation to thinking like autistic disorder, and abstract thinking. So, a nurse must be aware about different kind of thought process and should use this knowledge while providing care to their patient in hospital setting.

Suggested Reading

- Babu S. Psychology for Nurses. New Delhi, Elsevier Publication, 2014.
- Bhatia BD, Craig M. Elements of Psychology and Mental Health, 1st edn. Hyderabad, Orient Longman, 2006.
- Morgan CT, King RA, Weiz JR, et al. Introduction to Psychology, 7th edn. New Delhi. Tata McGraw Hill Publishing Company Ltd, 2007.
- Plotnik R. Introduction to Psychology, 5th edn. USA, Wadsworth Publishing Company, 1999.

REVIEW QUESTIONS

SHORT-ESSAY TYPE QUESTIONS

1. Define thinking and factors influencing thinking process.
2. Define types and level of thinking.

MULTIPLE CHOICE QUESTIONS

1. Deriving a specific conclusion from a universal statement is called:
   a. Inductive reasoning
   b. Deductive reasoning
   c. Concept
   d. Problem solving
2. Which is the highest level of thinking?
   a. Application
   b. Analysis
   c. Synthesis
   d. Evaluation

3. The generalized ideas about object or event, i.e. mentally conceived is called:
   a. Reasoning
   b. Thinking
   c. Problem solving
   d. Concept
4. Which of the following is not a building block of thinking?
   a. Concept
   b. Image
   c. Language
   d. Creativity
5. It is a kind of thinking in which an individual think for a problem on different point or angle and try to converge those ideas into one common ground in order to find a solution for the problem:
   a. Convergent thinking
   b. Critical thinking
   c. Divergent thinking
   d. Positive thinking
6. It is a type of thinking which start from part to whole or specific to general to find solution to a problem:
   a. Convergent thinking
   b. Critical thinking
   c. Inductive thinking
   d. Deductive thinking
7. It is a type of thinking in which thinking process involves a combination of positive and negative thoughts for someone or something:
   a. Convergent thinking
   b. Critical thinking
   c. Inductive thinking
   d. Deductive thinking

ANSWER KEY

1.	b	2.	d	3.	d	4.	c	5.	a	6.	c	7.	b

Chapter 7

Intelligence and Aptitude

INTRODUCTION

No two individuals are exactly alike. Some are bright, others dull, some are quick, others slow, some solve problems quickly and directly, others fumble over them for a long time, some adjust to new situation very easily and some take time and some time not able to adjust even. So how was it possible? It is because of individual difference. The teacher should conscious that there is individual difference in intelligence. The modern psychologist pays utmost attention to these individual differences.

NATURE AND MEANING OF INTELLIGENCE

There is no agreement as regards to exact definition and nature of intelligence. Many psychologists defined intelligence in their own ways. These definitions can be divided in following three groups.

1. **Ability to adjust:** This group of psychologists considered that intelligence is the ability to adjust to new environment. In this context many definitions are given.

'It is the capacity of flexible adjustment.' (Burt)

'Conscious adaptation to new situation is intelligence.' (Ross)

'Intelligence is the ability to adjust oneself to new situation.' (Stern)

'Intelligence means intellect put to use. It is the use of intellectual abilities for handling a situation or accomplishing any task.' (Woodworth)

2. **Ability to learn:** This group experts view intelligence as the capacity to learn. Some definition of this group experts are given here.

'Intelligence is the ability to learn.' (Buckingham)

'Intelligence is the ability to make profitable use of past experiences.' (Thorndike)

3. **Ability to carry abstract thinking:** According to this group's experts, intelligence is the ability to carry on abstract thinking

'Intelligence is the rational thinking.' (Spearman)

'Intelligence is a capacity to think well, to judge well and to be self-critical.' (Binet)

CHARACTERISTICS OF INTELLIGENCE

- Intelligence is an innate natural power and not acquired
- Power of intelligence differ from individual-to-individual
- It helps an a individual to learn new things and making adjustment
- It helps the individual to face and solve the difficult situation
- Hereditary determine and influence level of intelligence
- Environment, teaching and education affect intelligence
- Social, economic and cultural factors as well racial different effect on intelligence test score
- Gender is not a intenalable factor to determine intelligence
- IQ test proved an average level of IQ in children
- Development of intelligence ceases towards the middle of adolescence
- There is close relationship between intelligence and knowledge.

THEORIES OF INTELLIGENCE

There are various theories given by psychologist but none of them is complete one. To explain true nature of intelligence, psychologist put forward many theories. These different theories are:

1. Unitary or Monarchic Theory

Johnson and Stern were exponent of this theory. According to this theory, intelligence is the sum total of all human capabilities. It is power of energy which affects all activities of the individual.

Limitations

According to this theory, a man intelligent in doing one task will also intelligent in doing other as well as intelligence is the all round capacity of the individual.

For example, Dr APJ Abdul Kalam was a great scientist of India. According to this theory he could be a great artist if he wishes, but this was not true for him.

2. Primary Mental Ability Theory

Prof Thomson was exponent of this theory. This theory also known as sampling theory. The theory believes that intellectual abilities belong to certain groups which are not related to each other. Every group has prime factor. These primary abilities work independently of each other. These are nine groups of abilities according to this theory.

1. Visual or spatial ability
2. Perceptual
3. Numerical
4. Verbal comprehension
5. Word fluency
6. Memory
7. Inductive reasoning
8. Deductive reasoning
9. Problem solving.

So, according to this theory a child who is intelligent in group of knowledge may not be intelligent in other group. For example, a student intelligent in science subject may not be intelligent in mathematics.

3. Multiple Factor Theory

The exponent of this theory was Thorndike. According to this, intelligence is composed of highly particularized and independent faculties. There is no significant relation between them. According to this theory, we cannot infer the ability of a man in one sphere to his ability to another kind of work. For example, a student intelligent in mathematics would not give any clue to be intelligent in social sciences.

4. Eclectic or Two Factor Theory

Karl Pearson (1904) was the exponent of this theory. According to this theory, intelligence consist of two factors—one is 'g' factor and other is 's' factor. The 'g' factor is responsible for general ability and 's' factor stand for specific ability. Every individual has 'g' factor and some's' factors (or specific abilities). The factor 'g' is common in all individual but 's' factor vary from individual-to-individual. For doing any activity 'g' factor is always involved and some of the 's' factors are involved.

Some tasks require more of 'g' factors and other tasks require more of 's' factors. For example, solving a mathematical problem need more of 'g' factors whereas factors 's' is more needed for painting and playing piano. So factors 'g' remains the same and unchanged for an individual while 's' factors varies from task-to-task.

5. Triarchic or Three Factor Theory

This theory was proposed by Sternberg in 1988. According to this theory, intelligence is a decomposition of three factors/aspects; analytical, creative and practical. Analytical intelligence helps to sort out the problem by breaking the large problem in small parts. Creative intelligence helps to find new ways to solve a problem. Practical intelligence is the ability to use information to get along in life.

6. Fluid and Crystalloid Theory

Cattle was the founder of this theory. He said that intelligence is composed of two parts—i. fluid intelligence and ii. crystalloid intelligence. He also used general ability factors and put emphasis upon general or inherited potentialities and environmental factors. The earlier one was fluid and later one was crystalloid.

7. Theory of Primary Mental Abilities (Thurstone's Theory)

States that intelligent activities are neither an expression of innumerable highly specific factors, nor a general factor that pervades all mental activities. It is the essence of intelligence, as Spearman held. Instead, the analysis of interpretation of Spearman and others led them to the conclusion that 'certain' mental operations have in common a 'primary' factor that gives them psychological and functional unity and that differentiates them from other mental operations. These mental operations then constitute a group. A second group of mental operation has its own unifying primary factor, and so on. In other words, there are a number of groups of mental abilities, each of which has its own primary factor, giving the group a functional unity and cohesiveness.

Each of these primary factors is said to be relatively independent of the others. Thurstone has given the following six primary factors:

1. **The Number Factor (N):** Ability to do Numerical Calculations rapidly and accurately.
2. **The Verbal Factor (V):** Found in tests involving Verbal Comprehension.
3. **The Space Factor (S):** Involved in any task in which the subject manipulates the imaginary object in space.
4. **Memory (M):** Involving ability to memorize quickly.
5. **The Word Fluency Factor (W):** Involved whenever the subject is asked to think of isolated words at a rapid rate.
6. **The Reasoning Factor (R):** Found in tasks that require a subject to discover a rule or principle involved in a series or groups of letters. Based on these factors Thurstone constructed a new test of intelligence known as 'Test of Primary Mental Abilities (PMA).'

EMOTIONAL INTELLIGENCE (EI)

The term emotional intelligence has been in use since mid 20th century. The word emotional intelligence was first used in literacy criticism and psychiatry. This term has received a great deal of attention in the applied psychology and popular press.

NATURE AND MEANING OF EMOTIONAL INTELLIGENCE

The EI was first introduced by Salovey and Mayer (1990) and later expended by Goleman (1995). Emotional intelligence is the awareness and ability to manage one's own emotions as well as ability to be self-motivated, to feel what others feel and to be socially skilled. Emotional intelligence is a more powerful influence on success in life than more traditional views of intelligence. EI describes people's ability to perceive, understand and regulate their emotions.

Definition

'Emotional intelligence is the ability to perceive and express emotion; assimilate emotion in thought, understand and reason with emotion, and regulate emotion in self and others' (Mayer and Salovey, 1997).

'Emotional intelligence is a cognitive ability that involves the processing of emotion'.

It is also defined in term of behavior and skills including stress management (e.g. stress tolerance and impulse control), self-management skills (e.g. self-control, consciousness and adaptability) as well as social skills (e.g. conflict management, leadership and communication). A person with sound emotional intelligence may able to deal anger, impulsivity and anxiety in a rational way.

INTELLIGENT QUOTIENT (IQ, MENTAL RATIO)

The IQ was first introduced by Wilhelm Stern, a German Psychologist in 1912. In 1916, the idea of IQ was utilized in Stanford-Binet test. IQ is an index of intelligence. It is the ratio between mental age (MA) and chronological age (CA). By mental age we mean age perceived on the test and by chronological age we mean the real or actual age.

Formula for IQ

$$\text{IQ} = \frac{\text{Mental age (MA)}}{\text{Chronological age (CA)}} \times 100$$

For example, a 10-year-old child possesses the IQ of (MA) 5 years of his age. Thus his IQ is

$$\text{IQ} = \frac{5}{10} \times 100 = 50$$

So the IQ level of this child is 50.

Classification Based on IQ

Garrett, a great psychologist classified people according to their IQ in his book *'Great Experiments in Psychology'* as below.

IQ	Type
130 and above	Very superior
120–129	Superior
110–119	Bright normal
85–109	Average
70–84	Borderline
55–69	Mild mental retardation
40–54	Moderate mental retardation
25–39	Severe mental retardation

MEASUREMENT OF INTELLIGENCE

Psychologists invented many intelligence tests for children as well as adults. Broadly, the intelligence tests are classified under following ways:

Individual Tests

Individual tests are administered to individual. They are made to test the intelligence of individual. This test is again divided into two types: i. Verbal individual intelligence test and ii. Non-verbal individual intelligence test.

- **Verbal individual intelligence tests:** Verbal intelligence test use language. Some of popular test are discussed here.
  - **Binet Simon test:** Binet and Simon in 1905 published a scale of intelligence test. This scale consists of 30 different tasks from the simplest to the most complex in a serial order. This scale is prepared to test feeble minded children for age group 3–15 years. This scale extensively used almost all the European countries, America, Canada, Australia, New Zealand, South Africa, China, Japan, and Russia.
  - **Stanford Binet test (1916):** In 1916, Terman of Stanford University revised Binet test of intelligence. This revision was called Stanford Binet test. Terman made certain modification in Binet's test.
    - **Terman-Merril revision:** In 1937, Terman revised the Stanford Binet test with the help of Merril and published it. It was a useful intelligence test for children age group 2–18 years.
- **Non-verbal intelligence tests:** To overcome the limitation of verbal test for illiterate population non-verbal intelligence test was revised. Illiterate individuals are tested with the help of non-verbal individual intelligence tests. Some of the non-verbal test are explained here:
  - Pinter-Patterson performance scale
  - The Minnesota preschool scale
  - Arthur point scale of performance tests
  - Wechsler intelligence scale (mixed test—verbal and non-verbal)
  - Porteus Maze test
  - Gesell development schedule.

Group Intelligence Tests

As the name suggests these tests are designed to measure the intelligence of a group of people. All the people in a group are given same direction to perform for a given test. These tests are again classified:

- Verbal group tests
  - Army alpha test
  - Army general classification tests
  - Terman group test for mental ability.
- Non-verbal group tests (performance)
  - Army beta test
  - Raven's progressive matrix scale
  - Cattell's culture-free test.

Factors Influencing Intelligence

Every individual is unique in nature but differ in intelligence. Some people understand quickly and some learn very slowly. Psychologists believe that there are many factors which may influence intelligence level. Some factors are discussed here:

- **Education and training:** It has been evidenced that right education and appropriate training enhance intelligence level.
- **Socioeconomic and cultural barriers:** It is evidenced that person belong to poor socioeconomic status and bound to cultural barriers do not get higher score on intelligence test.
- **Environment:** It is one of the basic factors that influence intelligence level. It is been seen that children who are nurtured in good family environment have higher score on intelligence tests.
- **Hereditary:** The level of intelligence determined by the genes transmitted from his parents.
- **Physical health:** A good physical structure and health is a basic necessity for a sound for high level of intelligence. Ancient proverb, 'a sound mind lives in a sound body' justifies the importance of physical health for intelligence level.
- **Habitat:** It has seen that children belong to urban population have a higher intelligence level than rural habitat. It may be due to exposure of certain different types of environment and advance facilities.
- **Occupational status:** Many investigations proved that there is close relationship between occupation and intelligence level. Army alpha test indicate that engineers, lawyers, teachers, doctors and business executives obtained higher score on intelligence test than bookkeepers, photographers and policemen.

Use of Intelligence Tests

Intelligence tests are widely used nowadays in various fields in recruitment, selection, performance evaluation, promotion, demotion, for employers and students as well. Intelligence tests are useful in following ways:

Educational Uses

- Selection of courses
- Selection of pupil to school
- Classification of pupil
- Detection of various type of pupil
- Award of scholarship
- Promotion of pupil
- Prediction of success
- Assessment of teacher's work
- Evaluation of instructional material and methods
- Educational guidance.

Use in Vocational Guidance

Intelligence tests are used to guide for choosing the right vocation for an individual.

Use in Army and Civil Services

Selection in army and civil services, army officers all based on IQ testing.

Use in Research

To assign research work.

Use in Industry

Selection, promotion and performance.

Use in the Study of National and Racial Differences

With the help of IQ level of various races and nationalities can be identified.

Limitations of Intelligence Tests

- **Intelligence tests are not reliable:** Sometime intelligence test do not measures the exact IQ level of individual.
- **Intelligence tests are not accurate:** IQ test only contains certain limited number of items. It is a very crude method to assess IQ by using only a limited number of items related to selected fields.

- Intelligence tests are culture bound. So application is limited.
- IQ test tend to discriminate the child. Once the teacher came to know the IQ of a child. He will consider or see the child on the level of IQ level. So intelligence test discriminate a child by labeling him.
- There is shortage of intelligence test. This tends to limit the scope of assessment of child's future limited to only selected areas.

INTELLIGENCE AND SICKNESS

A healthy mind lives in a healthy body inferred the relationship of health and intelligence. A low level of intelligence itself indicates a sickness or morbidity. For example, mental retarded and feeble mind children are always a serious challenge for medical sciences. In every sphere of life, mental retarded children find challenges and find unable to compete with others. Mental retardation is considered a disorder by American Psychiatric Association and DSM IV classification.

Although, there is no direct relation of intelligence of sickness with intelligence but anxiety and fear related to sickness may have negative impact on intelligence. However, this relation is limited to physical disorders only and in some psychological disorders, i.e. Down syndrome, and Parkinsonism, the level of intelligence will be declined. In case of severe psychotic disorder, i.e. schizophrenia, the level of cognitive function is grossly disorganized and predispose declination in intelligence level. However, sometimes disorganization of cognitive features helps the patient to use intelligence in wrong ways, i.e. psychopathic personality disorder patient has intact cognitive functions but they use intelligence to do crime.

A subnormal level of intelligence results into various problem during sickness, i.e. understanding the nature of disease, compliance to drugs, showing uncooperative behavior and importance of diet and nutrition, etc. Failure to compliance to treatment ultimately results to slow down the recovery process.

INTELLIGENCE AND NURSING

Intelligence is crucial for success in every sphere of nursing. The nursing job is full of challenges and unpredictable. A nurse meets with different types of patients in day-to-day life and need decision to meet the care accordingly. So, an intelligent nurse is able to analyze the situation and can quickly respond to it. Adjustment with hospital and its related department is another challenging job for a nurse. A well intelligent nurse know various methods to get adjust with the situation and can adjust to it. However, it is also important for an intelligent nurse to meet and help different kind of relatives, family friends and other well wishes to make adjust with the situation.

APTITUDE

Introduction

Aptitude has been observed in the individuals that differ from one another and within themselves in one or the other filed of activity such as dance, music, art and mechanical job, etc. If we observe human life no one is perfect to perform all activities for example, a dance teacher teaches dance to all his students but only few students able to perform in a perfect manner than others. Such students are said to possess certain specific abilities other than intelligence which help them in achieving success in some particular areas or activities (i.e. occupation, education, etc). These specific abilities are known as aptitude.

Generally, many people use the terms aptitude and intelligence interchangeably. To clear it, aptitude may be considered as a specific ability or specific capacity besides the general intelligence ability that helps individual to acquire a required degree of proficiency or achievement in a specific field.

Meaning and Definition of Aptitude

An aptitude is a person's special ability, or in other words, his inherent skills. Aptitude usually refers to a collection of abilities which happen to be of value in a particular culture. Different psychologists define aptitude in their own manner.

'Aptitude refers to those qualities characterizing a person's way of behavior that serve to indicate how well we can learn to meet and solve certain specific kind of problems.' (Bingham, 1937)

'An aptitude is a present condition which indicates an individual's potentialities for future.' (Traxler, 1957)

'Aptitude is a combination of characteristics indicate of an individual's capacity to acquire (with training) some specific knowledge, skills or set of organized responses such as the ability to speak a language, to become a musician, to do a mechanical work, etc.' (Freeman, 1971)

So, we can say that aptitude is a specific ability or capacity of an individual to acquire proficiency in the specific area of learning.

Classification of Aptitude

An individual capable to perform different kind of activities, therefore the abilities to produce specific abilities are also limitless. However, the aptitude classified under following headings.

- **Sensory aptitude:** It includes all those aptitudes that are related to sensory capacities like hearing, taste, touch, smell, sense of sight, etc.
- **Mechanical aptitude:** This aptitude concerned with the ability to deals with various mechanical devices and gadgets, i.e. flying aero plane, driving formula motor racing car, etc.
- **Artistic aptitude:** It is all the related to the expression of artistic abilities and expression, i.e. writing, painting, music and designing, etc.
- **Professional aptitude:** This abilities concerned with activities of various profession and occupations, i.e. clerical aptitude, criminal aptitude, legal aptitude, nursing aptitude, pilot aptitude and engineering aptitude, etc.
- **Scholastic aptitude:** This aptitude concerned to academic performance and achievements, i.e. scientific aptitude, medical aptitude, commercial aptitude, sport aptitude, linguistic aptitude, etc.

Measurement of Aptitude

Like intelligence various types of aptitudes tests are available to measure the aptitude to predict the area of interest and future success of an individual. Broadly, these aptitude test classified under following headings.

General Aptitude Tests

General aptitude tests use batteries to measure the achievement and performance of an individual form particular area. There are two major general aptitude tests.

- **General aptitude test battery (GATB):** GATB developed by the employment service Bureau of the United State, which contain 12 tests. In this battery, 8 tests are paper-pencil test, which includes comparison, computation, vocabulary, arithmetic, reasoning, form matching, test matching and three-dimensional matching. The other four tests are performance based such as assembling and dissembling rivets and washers, etc. This test measures the abilities such as general intelligence, verbal aptitude, numerical aptitude, spatial aptitude, form perception, clerical aptitude, motor coordination, finger dexterity and manual dexterity.

- **Differential aptitude test (DAT):** DAT developed by Psychological Corporation of United States. It includes test for verbal reasoning, numerical ability, abstract reasoning, spatial relation, mechanical reasoning, clerical speed, accuracy and two test for language-spelling and grammar.

Specific Aptitude Tests

These tests are developed to assess the specific abilities in a particular area. These tests are classified as follows:

- **Mechanical aptitude tests:** These tests include abilities like sensory and motor abilities, perception of spatial relationship, ability to understand mechanical fractions and mechanical relationship. Some well-known mechanical aptitude test name are given here.
  - Minnesota mechanical assembly test
  - Minnesota spatial relation test
  - Revised minnesota paper form board test
  - Bennett mechanical compression test.
- **Musical aptitude tests:** These aptitude tests developed to measure various aspects related to music like pitch, sound, rhythm, tone, intensity, etc. These tests developed to discover the musical talents.
- **Clerical aptitude tests:** These tests helps to know the job-related performance especially in clerical areas. Clerical aptitude test includes perceptual ability, language ability and motor ability. Some common clerical tests are given here.
  - Clerical aptitude test battery–Developed by Bureau of Educational and Vocational Guidance, Patna (Hindi and English)
  - Minnesota vocational tests for clerical workers
  - Detroit clerical aptitude examination.
- **Graphic art aptitude tests:** These tests are developed to discover the talent related to graphic art and design. Some common tests name are given here.
  - Home art aptitude inventory
  - Meier art judgment test.

- **Scholastic and professional aptitude tests:** These tests are developed to find scholastic and professional abilities related to study and job, i.e. teaching, learning, training, law, medicine, engineering, etc. Some common used tests name are given here.
  - Scientific aptitude test
  - Moss scholastic aptitude test (for medical students)
  - Tale legal aptitude test
  - Shah's teaching aptitude test
  - Pre-engineering ability aptitude test.

Use of Aptitude Tests

Aptitude tests are widely used in teaching, job, and training and almost in all areas. Some popular uses of aptitude tests are given here.

- **Vocational and carrier guidance:** These tests are widely used for guiding the students for specific course and filed of vocation.
- **Selection of candidates:** These tests are used for selection of suitable students for educational and professional courses and vocation as well.
- **Uses in nursing:** Nursing aptitude tests are helpful in prediction of professional skills related to the area of specialization.

Suggested Reading

- Butcher HJ. Human Intelligence and Its Nature and Assessment. London: Methun & Co, 1968.
- Chaplin Jamesh P, Krawiec TS. Systems and Theories of Psychology. New York: Holt Rinehart & Winston Inc, 1974.
- Goleman D. Emotional Intelligence. New York: Bantam, 1995.
- Guilford JP. The Nature of Human Intelligence. New York: McGraw Hill Book Co, 1957.
- Smith Wendell. Conditioning and Instrumental Learning. McGraw Hill, 1966.
- Sternberg RJ. The Triarchic Mind: A New Theory of Human Intelligence. New York: Viking Penguin, 1988.
- Stoddard GD. The Meaning of Intelligence. New York: Macmillan, 1943.

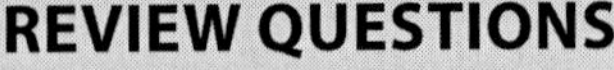

REVIEW QUESTIONS

SHORT-ESSAY TYPE QUESTIONS

1. Define intelligence and discuss factors affecting intelligence.
2. Enlist various theories of intelligence and discuss any one theory in detail.
3. Define emotional intelligence and its uses.
4. Discuss various types of intelligence test, its advantages and disadvantages.
5. Define aptitude, its types and use of aptitude tests.

MULTIPLE CHOICE QUESTIONS

1. The normal IQ is:
   a. 90-110
   b. 70-90
   c. 50-70
   d. < 50
2. Which of the following intelligence test is revised and translated to Indian population?
   a. Wechsler adult intelligence test
   b. Stanford-Binet intelligence scale
   c. Alexander pass along tests
   d. Koh's Block design test
3. Which of the following intelligence test is not a example of verbal intelligence test?
   a. Army alpha
   b. Alexander pass along test
   c. Army general classification test
   d. Stanford Binet Scale of Intelligence
4. The mental ability which is commonly used to all forms of intellectual activity is called:
   a. Group intelligence
   b. Multiple intelligence
   c. Specific mental ability
   d. General mental ability
5. Who has given the term Intelligence quotient (IQ)?
   a. Alfred Binlet
   b. EL Thorndike
   c. David Wechsler
   d. William Stern
6. Who is the father of intelligence test construction?
   a. Guilford
   b. LL Thurston
   c. Alfred Binet
   d. Sternberg

7. Which of the following psychologist stated that intelligence has 150 factors?
   a. Alfred Binet
   b. EL Thorndike
   c. David Wechsler
   d. Guilford
8. Which of the following activities is not related to bodily kinesthetic intelligence?
   a. Gymnastics
   b. Navigation
   c. Surgery
   d. Dancing
9. Single factor theory of intelligence was given by ________
   a. Alfred Binet
   b. Thorndike
   c. Freeman
   d. None of them
10. Who is the father of theory of multiple intelligence?
   a. Gardner
   b. Piaget
   c. Brunner
   d. Vroom

ANSWER KEY

1.	a	2.	b	3.	b	4.	d	5.	d	6.	c	7.	d
8.	b	9.	a	10.	a								

Chapter 8

Motivation and Emotion

INTRODUCTION

Motivation is an important concept in understanding the behavior of the individual. It includes numerous complex aspect of human behavior to which contribution has been made by various professionals in which psychologists come first. It refers to the basic questions, 'why an individual does what he does', why some people perform well, while others do not?' answer of all these questions lies in the concept of motivation. Motivation can be defined as those forces within an individual that push or propel him to satisfy basic needs or want (York, 1976). Abraham Maslow said that only satisfied need provide the source of motivation; a unsatisfied need create no tension and therefore no motivation.

MEANING AND DEFINITION OF MOTIVATION

A motive is what prompts a person to act in a certain way or at least develop on inclination for specific behavior. Motivation generated from the Latin word *'movere'* which means 'to move'. Thus, in literal language we can say that motivation is the process of arousing movement in the organism. Motivation has been defined by various psychologists in various ways.

'Motivation refers to arousal of tendency to act to produce one or more effect.' (Atkinson)

'Motivation is the process of arousing action, sustain the activity in progress and regulating the pattern of activity.' (PT Young)

'Motivation refers to the way in which urges, desires, aspiration drives, strivings, needs direct control or explain the behavior of human being.' (Dalson)

'Motivation is a constant, never ending fluctuation and complex phenomena and it is an almost universal characteristics of every organism.' (AbrahamMaslow)

'Motivation refers to existence of an organism faced sequence, to its direction and content and its persistence in given direction or stability of content.' (DO Hebb)

It is common that three qualities are included in most definitions, a) it is presumed internal force, b) that energizes for action, and c) determine the direction of action.

Thus, far motivational process has been viewed as a decision making process which takes place within the employees.

NATURE OF MOTIVES

- Motivation is an inner state or an aroused feelings
- It compels an individual to attain the target by buildup tension or urges to act
- It is goal-directed activity that energizes an individual to attain goal
- Attainment of goal helps in the releases of tension aroused by specific motives
- A change in goal may leads to change in nature and degree of motivation.

FUNCTIONS OF MOTIVATION

Many psychologists analyzed the motivated behavior of an organism and observe the following functions of motivated behavior.

- **Motives energies and sustain behavior:** Motives always give energy to the behavior of an organism and arouse him for action. The energy can be physiological as in drives that are emotionally the energy can be physiological for emotional significant drives of human being. The energy is supplied in the proportion to the amount of energy needed for completion of task. A motive not only gives energy for completion of task but also sustain interest and attention for long period to complete that task.
- **Motives direct and regulate our behavior:** Motivated state is often described as guided, directed and goal-oriented. The motivated behavior moves in a specific direction. The behavior of an organism is purposeful and persistent. The direction of motivational behavior is very complex because of the structure of situation and the action sequences which determine the behavior.
- **Motivation always makes behavior selective:** Under motivational conditions the behavior of the organism does not move

in haphazard way. It is directed towards a selected goal which the individual set for himself or herself, e.g. the students who is motivated to secure high grade in the examination concentrates on his studies by selecting appropriate means to reach on his preselected goal, i.e. securing high grade.

MOTIVATIONAL CYCLES OR SEQUENCE

Most of our motives have a psychic nature, i.e. they originate from some need either physiological or psychological. The need create a drive state in organism that push the organism to behave in a certain fashion to satisfy the need. It is called motivational cycle. A motivational cycle has following elements—need, drive, incentive and goal.

Need

A need involves an organism desire or wants or demand. This condition of demand makes the organism to seek particular goal or end state. This goal can be an object or a person from the environment or an inner condition, i.e. satisfaction. A need may be biological and psychological which may arise with or without deprivation. So, it can be said that need is a generalize condition of desire and want which direct an individual to identify a particular goal and direct his activities to fulfill it.

Types of Needs (Fig. 8.1)

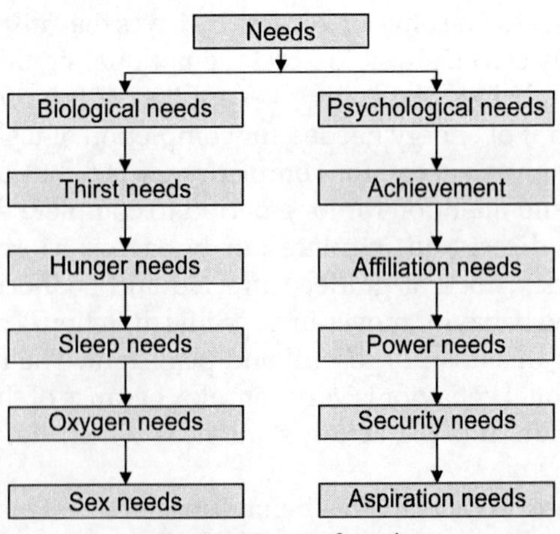

Fig. 8.1: Types of needs

Drive

It is a hypothetical condition and a force which impels or pushes a person or animal to achieve the defined goal. It cannot be observed but it can be inferred from behavior. The concept of drive takes two basic characteristics of a motivated behavior (Fig. 8.2). There are:

- Whenever an organism is under a motivated condition there is an increased activity.
- This increased activity sooner or later comes to an end when the condition which caused the increased activity are removed, eliminated or goal is achieved.

For example, a person is hungry and wants to eat something immediately. Now, the person starts searching some place like restaurant, or hotel to take food. Here, the hunger is need of person and the force which compels the person to search the food to satisfy hunger is called drive.

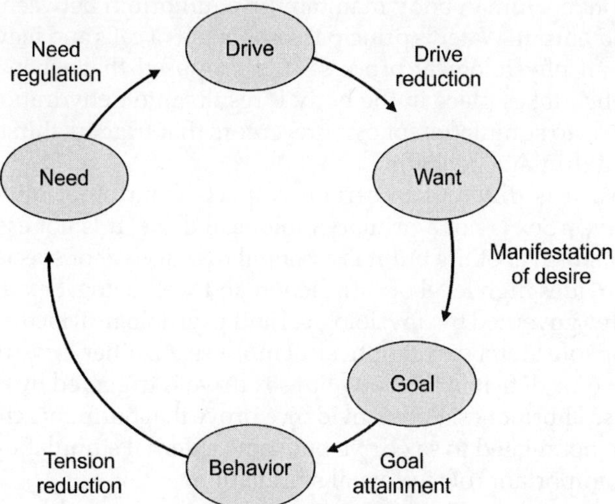

Fig. 8.2: Motivation cycle

Incentive and Goal

The concept of incentive is closely related to drive, e.g. if a person has a hunger need and he wish to eat but he realizes that the food which he has been served, he does not like, then he might suddenly feels that he is no longer hungry and vice versa. Incentive can be positive or negative.

TYPES OF MOTIVATION

Broadly motivation is classified under following two headings:

Physiological or Primary Motives

Physiological motives also known as biological motives. These include hunger, sex, thirst, the need of rest, sleep and elimination needs.

- **Hunger motive:** This is most primitive and dominant motive in human being. Earlier, it was believed that contractions in the stomach develop the drive of hunger. However, in certain experiment on rats when stomach was removed hunger was still experienced. Many other scientific views that lowering blood glucose, metabolic changes triggers hunger drive.
- **Thirst:** Local stimulus theory (LST) states that dryness of lips triggers thirst drive but it cannot be a strong factor to regulate high drinking behavior. It is found to be stronger than hunger motive. Human body maintaining equilibrium between input and output. Water is principal component of cells and inevitable to all physiological process. It is proposed that when water deficit takes place in the body it results into dehydration that leads to stimulation of osmoreceptors that triggers thirst drive and drinking behavior.
- **Sex:** It is different in certain respects from other biological drives. Sex is not a primary biological drive. It is not essential for survival of life but it is essential for survival of species and provides high level of satisfaction and well-being. Sex drive is often governed by physiological and psychological factors, thus it is considered psychophysical motives. As other drive related to some deficit in the body but sex drive is triggered by release of sex hormones. Recent evidence prove that hormonal changes are not related to sex drive but some external stimulation play an important role in sexual stimulation.
- **Rest and sleep:** Need for sleep and rest is one more physiological motives. When body systems works for very long time without sleep and rest, it is possible to experience fatigue and tiredness. Hence, the body demand rest and sleep.
- **Need of elimination of waste:** Elimination need is strong as other needs. When the body cavities, i.e. bladder and bowel become distended with waste material, they cause pressure and discomfort. This discomfort and pressure lead restless and urge to pass urine and stool.

- **Need of oxygen:** Need of oxygen is the most prime and essential physiological need since conception to till death. Nerve and heart cells are sensitive to oxygen deprivation and deficiency leads to severe degeneration of cells. Oxygen must be delivered from environment to lung, purified and supplied to body tissues.

Social or Secondary Motives

Social motives are important for existence in a society. These are those motives which a child learns in society during development. These motives are differing to biological motives in not having cyclic pattern. Social motives differ in degree in different individuals. Social motives include achievement, affiliation, power and need for status.

- **The need of achievement:** Achievement motivation refers to a drive towards some standard of excellence. High achievers challenge failure and work harder while low achievers accept failure and go for easy task. Children whose family condition and parents have accepted their independence tend to become higher achievers. It is the achievement motivation, which refers to the desire of a person to meet standard of excellence. Need of achievement influence the perception of situation and goal setting. According to McClelland, people with higher achievement have certain characteristic like preoccupation with task, accomplishment, feedback and taking risk.
- **Affiliation motives:** Man is a social being and cannot exist in isolation. The affiliation needs seen fulfilled by attachment with others through friendship, sociability and group membership. Seeking other people fellow being and wanting to be close to them, both physically and psychologically is affiliation. It is a desire of human being to be associated with others, to be in company, to touch, to feel and to think as often do. The affiliation motive gives feeling of social security.
- **Power motives:** Power is defined as the capacity or ability of a person to produce intended effect on the behavior or emotions on others. Person with higher power will be dominant and ruled the weaker section of the society. Power is exercised by joining club, political parties, organizations, and association. Powerful person often try to convince other with the help of power, engage in more competitive games and drink more

heavily. Power motives also observed in animals and birds, i.e. power made lion a king of jungle.

- **Need of status:** Everyone wish to stand independently among the people or society and want an individualized image in the eye of others. Need of status is also observed in animal and birds.
- **Aggression motives:** Human aggression encompass all behavior that is intended to inflict physical and psychological harm on other. Long time intense frustration, anxiety and conflict can trigger anxiety. Mass media playing an important role model to instigate aggressive behavior in human.

THEORIES OF MOTIVATION

Various psychologists have proposed many theories to clear the concept of motivation. Some of the important theories are discussed here.

Physiological Theory

Physiological theory was proposed by Morgan and it is also known as central motive state (CMS) theory. He believed that there is a central motive state which is the basis of all activities and behaviors. Morgan conducted several experiments and gathered evidences in support of his theory. He mentioned following characteristics of central motive state theory.

- **Persistent:** A CMS when once aroused remains persistent and does not require support from any other internal or external stimulants.
- **General activity:** The motivated organism has increased bodily activity.
- **Selectivity:** A CMS results in selectivity of reaction to stimuli. The reaction does not depend on any external environmental stimuli.
- **Omission of certain behavior:** The most significant CMS is that it prompts the organism for appropriate customary behavior.

In order to substantiate theory Morgan has conducted a number of neurophysiological studies and experiments to support the view of CMS. Theory limitation lies in that it is hypothetical concept which is not an anatomical structure which deals with motivated behavior.

Maslow Theory

Theory of self-actualization was developed by Abraham Maslow whose approach to understand human personality was different from behaviorist and psychoanalyst. He has consistently argued that needs are arranged in a hierarchical order. He said that, 'as one general type of need is satisfied another higher order need will emerge and become operative in life'. Maslow has developed a hierarchical order of need from physiological to self-actualization of needs. The order of needs start from basic survival or lower needs to higher order needs. The hierarchic is as follow (Fig. 8.3).

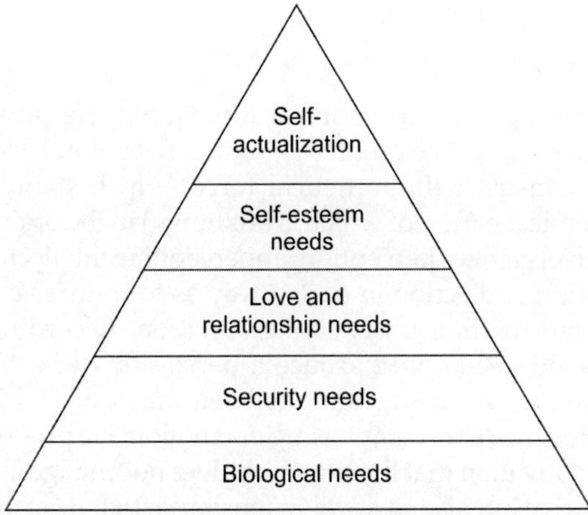

Fig. 8.3: Maslow's needs hierarchy

- **Biological needs:** Biological need is the most important need of human being. According to Maslow when this need is deprived for longer period, all other needs fail to appear in the background.
- **Safety needs:** When the biological needs are successfully fulfilled, then safety needs become the dominant force in the personality of individual. Safety needs are many are mainly concerned with maintaining order and security.
- **Love and belongingness:** The need at this category emphasizes the basic psychological nature of human being to identify group life. There are needs of making intimate relationship with other member of society. These needs are dependent on the fulfillment and satisfaction of previous needs.

- **Self-esteem:** Self-confidence and sense of self-worth
  - **Esteem from others:** Valuation of self from others
  - **Self-esteem:** Feeling of self-confidence and self-respect.
- **Self-actualization:** It is the highest need in hierarchical system proposed by Maslow. Self-actualization person wants to be free restrain from society. They demonstrate an efficient perception of reality and acceptance. They accept of self and others. They are democratic in outlook. They are having personality of problem centered orientation.

Need hierarchy based on the concept of 'prepotency' of needs. Prepotency defined as need emerges as a motivator after satisfying a lower (more prepotent) need.

Murray's Theory

Murray developed need theory of motivation. He puts forward the concept of need to explain the human behavior. He described need as a construct (hypothetical force) which stand for force (physiochemical nature of which is unknown) in the brain region, a force which organizes perception, apperception, intellectualization and condition and action in such a way as to transfer in a certain direction and existing unsatisfying situation. According to him, an unsatisfied need could arouse a person to work that would be sustained until satisfaction has been intended. Each need is accompanied by a particular feeling or emotion. He proposed in his theory of motivation that the organism does not engage in activities to reduce drive but also to develop tension so that it can be later on reduced. According to him tensionless state is not satisfying but the process at reducing tension satisfies the need. He classifies all the needs in two categories.

1. **Physical needs (primary needs):** Satisfaction of basic physiological process, i.e. hunger, thirst, sleep, rest, sex, elimination, etc. These needs are essential for survival of organism.
2. **Psychological needs (secondary needs):** These needs emerge out of primary needs. And concerned with emotional and mental satisfaction, i.e. needs for achievement, affiliation, aggression, autonomy and superiority.

Implications of Murray's Theory

- Helps to understand own and other behavior
- Needs vary in importance among people
- Direct people's behavior towards or away from the objects

- Helps to shape the motivated system
- Helps in understanding behavior we see every day.

ERG Theory of Motivation

CA Alberger (1961) was chief exponent of ERG (existence, relatedness and growth) theory. This theory is derived from Maslow's need theory. ERG mostly applied to the study of human motivation in the workplace as tool for increasing morale and productivity. He classified Maslow's five needs under three categories as follows:

1. **Existence needs:** Include all material and physiological needs, i.e. food, water, air, clothing, safety, love and affection, etc.
2. **Relatedness:** Encompass social and self-esteem needs and emphasizes the importance of relationship of friend, family, relatives and other in life of an individual.
3. **Growth need:** It is related to internal satisfaction and self-actualization. This needs impel a person to make creative or productive effect on him.

Herzberg's Two Factor Theory

It is also called Herzberg two factor theory of motivation. This theory focuses on some sources of motivation which are pertinent to accomplishment of a task. Herzberg concluded that job satisfaction and dissatisfaction was the product of two separate factors (Table 8.1).

1. Motivating factors (satisfiers)
2. Hygiene factors (dissatisfiers).

Table 8.1: Comparison of satisfiers and dissatisfiers

Satisfiers	Dissatisfiers
Achievement	Company policy
Recognition	Supervision
Work itself	Working condition
Responsibility	Interpersonal relationship
Advancement	Salary
Growth	Status
	Job security
	Personal life

Herzberg used the term 'hygiene' in medical sense—the sense that it operate to remove hazards from the environment. According to Herzberg theory, hygiene cannot motivate; and when used to achieve this goal it can actually produce negative effects over the long run. A hygiene environment prevents discontent with a job, but such as environment cannot lead the individual beyond a minimal adjustment consisting of the absence of dissatisfaction. A positive 'happiness' seems to require some attainment of psychological growth.

McClelland's Need for Achievement Theory

McClelland proposed a theory of motivation that is closely related to the concept of learning. This proposes that when a need is strong in a person, its effect is to motivate the person to use behavior which leads to satisfaction of the need. The main theme of McClelland theory is that needs is learned through coping with one's environment. Since needs are learned, behavior which is rewarded tend to recur at higher frequency. The need for achievement or nAch involves the desire to independently master object, idea and other people, to increase self-esteem through the exercise of one's talent. McClelland research indicates that individual motivation based on 3 needs. These are:

1. **Need for achievement (NAch):** The drive to excel, to achieve in relation to set standard, to strive to succeed.
2. **Need for power (NPower):** The need to make other behave in your own way.
3. **Need for affiliation (NAff):** The need for making friends, close relationship and intimacy.

METHODS TO MEASURE NEEDS/MOTIVES

It is very difficult to measures the human motivation because it is interrelated with several variables and moreover it becomes more problematic when motivation is partially conscious and partially unconscious. Although psychologist attempting to device methods of measuring human motivation and they have developed several method to measure human motivation in which few are described here.

- **Experimental method:** It is strictly confined to psychology laboratory to measure the motivation. Initially the experiments were conducted on animals and later on they were carried out on human beings. In these experiments human being were deprived for water and food for several hours and days to measure the strength thirst and hunger drive. Atkinson and McClelland conducted an experiment to study the hunger motives among hungry Navy personals that were deprived of food for 16 hours and a group of comparable subjects who were not deprived of food but were immediately introduced in experimental group after they had their meal. The story written by them in response to some pictures compared and great difference were found in their food imagination.

- **Self-rating technique:** This is the simplest and oldest technique of motives/need measurement. In this technique two procedures can be followed—i. Direct method—subject is asked to fill out a rating scale or a questionnaire, and ii. Indirect method—the subject is asked to indicate his likes or dislikes for a variety of activities ranging from objects to values. On the basis of his likes and dislikes strength of motives is determined. The first effort in this regard was made by Tylor in 1953 by developing an anxiety questionnaire as an indirect measure of drive strength.
- **Rating of motivation by observer (observation method):** Self-reporting technique have not been found so much reliable. So it was replaced by rating technique, in which motives are rated by other observers. This technique is most useful in exploring unconscious motives of which the subject himself is not aware.
- **Behavioral measure of motivation:** Behavioral measure detect the presence of motivation or motives by observing the response of the person under some conditions. Physiological responses, psychological learning, perception, coping behavior, expressive behavior may provide information of the motives of the person.
- **Projective techniques:** Projective techniques are also helpful to measure motives or motivation. There are few projective techniques by which we can measure the motivation.

  Thematic apperception test (TAT): In this test subjects are shown a series of ambiguous pictures and asked to narrate a story about what is going on each picture in their own words. The psychologist then identifies the needs being projected and judges from the number of related items in the story how strong each need is.

MOTIVATION AND HEALTH

Everyone have some motive in their life, someone want to become doctor, some want good husband someone want to become intelligent and many more. It would not be surprise if we give life and motivation is used synonymously. Now we can say that to live a good life, a tough physical health is needed and so for motivation. Deviation in health may decline motivation and losses of desire to live. For example, a severe depressive patient lost the hope for life and has suicidal thoughts. The person is having suicidal thoughts because he lost the hope for future life. So, loosing motives related to loosing mental as well as physical health of an individual.

In modern world of competition, a person should be motivated enough to achieve the goal for survival in life. There could be many barriers in between you and your target but the motivation should be keep on high for energizing yourself to achieve the desired goal.

MOTIVATION AND NURSING

Everyone needs motivation in life to perform certain tasks. This motivation could be in the form of reassurance, counseling, showing direction, money, support and many other forms. A nurse should also understand the need of motivation. He can motivate the behavior of a patient by encouraging, reassuring, showing positive aspects of life and value of life. Providing need-based motivation help the patient to become more cooperative and helping in recovery process. However, it is also big concern for a professional nurse to develop a motive to service the humanity. So, while selecting nursing as a carrier profession, she should understand the aspect of serving humanity in mind to keep his motive high. A high level of motivation helps to energizes to do the work with best interest.

EMOTION

The word emotion is derived from the Latin word 'Emovere' which means 'agitation or disturbed mind or excitement'. In simple way, emotion is a state of excitement or disturbance in mental and psychological functions. Usually, emotions are equated with feelings but there is a difference in feelings and emotions. In the words of Gates, 'emotions are episode in which the individual is moved or excited.'

DEFINITION OF EMOTION

'Emotion is 'moved' or 'stirred-up' state of an organism. It is stirred-up state of feeling that is the way it appears to the individual himself. It is the disturbed muscular and glandular activity that is the way, it appears to an external observer.' (Woodworth, 1945)

'Emotions are episodes in which the individual is moved or excited.' (Gates)

'Emotion is an acute disturbance of the individual as a whole psychological in origin, conscious experience and visceral functioning.' (PT Young)

CHARACTERISTICS OF EMOTIONS

- **Emotions are subjective in nature:** People react differently to different situation. Some people are very bold to certain deadly situation and can face but other cannot. Emotions are most personal and subjective cognitive phenomena of an individual.
- **Emotions are result of external stimulus:** An event or stimulus outside in environment may arouse the emotional state in an individual.
- **Emotions energize a person:** Sometimes, strong emotions give lot of energy and propel us to face the situation. For example, fear of losing a race may propel a person to run fast.
- **Emotions may be pleasant or painful:** Emotions may be pleasant or painful, i.e. joy, love, sorrow, crying, shouting, fear and anger, etc.
- **Emotions bring physiological and psychological changes:** It is well-understood phenomena that different emotions related to different physiological and psychological outcomes, e.g. fear leads to increase heart rate, sweating and sadness leads to decrease body responses.

TYPICAL EMOTIONS

Knowledge of common emotions will help us to understand their emotional behavior. This knowledge will help in dispelling the belief that the child who becomes emotionally aroused and behave in an unsocial way is an immature emotional. Moreover, this knowledge will give clues as to when expect different forms of emotional expressions. The common experienced emotions are as under:

- **Anger:** Anger is the one of the most common emotion in human beings as well as in animals. Both children and adult experience this emotion and it has higher impact on personality.

Anger is the outburst of chronic inner frustration and conflict. It can also predisposed by physical weakness, illness, hunger, fatigue and restlessness, unfulfilled dreams and wishes. Anger may be expressed in certain ways like shouting, laughing, crying, eye staring, kicking, and participating in certain competition.

- **Fear:** Like anger fear is another one of the basic emotions of human being. Since birth the children are more or less troubled by fear. With the development of intelligence the child start understanding many things and fear will be reduced automatically. Fear may be because of certain things like illness, immediate danger, overprotection, unpleasant experience of childhood, and watching and listening horrible stories, etc.
- **Happiness:** Happiness is another common emotion in human being. Healthy individuals are usually happy. If the individual possess good health he remains happy and cheerful. Happiness can be expressed by many ways, i.e. laughing, smiling, cheering, jumping up and down, roaring with open mouth, hugging, kissing and many more ways.
- **Affection:** Like happiness, affection is another pleasant emotion. It is similar to happiness in that it brings about a happy response. Affection is a pleasurable association with the person with whom they are more comfortable and able to fulfill all physical and psychological needs. Affection is not an innate emotional response. Affection is learned by many objects, persons and things as the child grow. Affection is expressed by hugging, kissing, founding, cuddling, and taking and meeting the needs of concerned one.
- **Curiosity:** Human being is curious by nature. He is eager to know about new and unusual things and events. Curiosity will help an individual to explore the surrounding and find new things and conditions in order to get adjustment and advancement in life.
- **Love:** Unlike to biological needs, love is also a basic necessity of human beings as well as of animals. Love can be expressed by many ways like hugging, kissing, founding, sympathy, showing affection and taking care of person.
- **Crying:** Crying is the first primitive emotion develops in newborn and human being. It is first ever emotion in a child to fulfill different needs like hunger and sleep.

PHYSIOLOGICAL CHANGES IN EMOTIONS

Emotions are always accompanied with strong physiological changes as follows:

- **Heartbeat:** Emotional changes are result in fluctuation in heartbeat. The fluctuation in heart can be measured by electrocardiogram (ECG).
- **Blood pressure:** Emotional excitement leads to changes in blood vessels by dilating and constructing blood vessels.
- **Respiratory rate:** Emotion also leads to variation in respiratory rate. It may rise and fall.
- **Pulse rate:** Changes in emotion lead to changes in pulse rate. In case of emotional excitement the pulse rate will be increased and vice versa.
- **Digestive system:** It is seen that temporary changes in emotional state lead to increase digestive functions and chronic emotional state leads to decrease and negative impact on digestive system, i.e. decreased absorption, frequent diarrhea, ulcerative colitis, peptic ulcer.
- **Effect on other systems:** Emotional state leads to changes in other bodily systems, i.e. increased sweating, salivation, increased urination, increase blood sugar, erect hair on the skin, dilation of pupil, muscular tension and tremors, etc.
- **Brain waves:** Alertness of brain is observed in the form of brain waves. In case relaxation and excitement the speed and various are noticed in brain waves.
- **Change in behavior:** Emotional state leads to changes in behavior or subjective expression. Emotional experience can be noticed by facial expressions, i.e. trembling of voice, high pitched loud voice, increase hand and feet movement, trembling voice, screaming, smiling face, laughing, and crying, etc.

THEORIES OF EMOTION

Many theorists proposed many theories of the emotions. Most of theories were based on mechanism of its origin and its experience at conscious and bodily level. Some theories are given below.

James Lang Theory

S William James proposed first theory of emotion in 1880s. A Danish Psychologist Carl Lange also gave the similar concept. According to this theory felt experience is the result of bodily changes. It is observed that emotional changes are the results of visceral and motor reactions in the bodily system and theses changes are interpreted in term of emotional feelings. For example, when we look a lion, we run first to avoid it, then notice our fear and trembling (Fig. 8.4).

Cannon-Bard Theory

Exponents of this theory were Walter Cannon and Philip Bard (1920s). This theory said that bodily changes and emotional experience occurs at same time. An emotional experience is activated by the external inputs to the sensory organs. When we see or hear stimuli, the nervous system activated immediately and we express emotionally. For example, on confronting a wild dog, the running and feeling of fear will take place at the same time.

According to this theory as soon as the stimulation reaches to thalamus and cortex, the emotional experience perceived and felt; it does not depends upon the feedback from internal organs and skeleton responses.

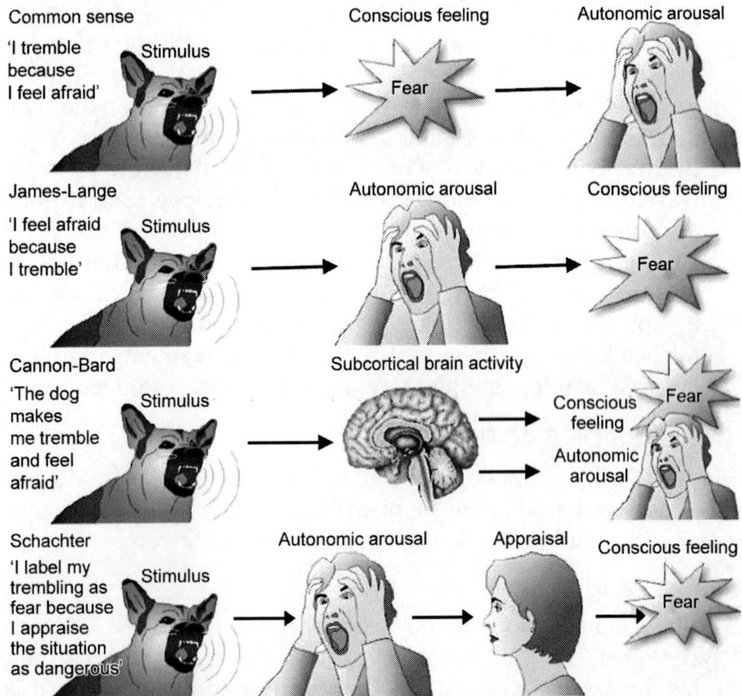

Fig. 8.4: James-Lange and Cannon-Bard theory concept

Schachter-Singer Theory

This theory also known as cognitive arousal theory of emotions. This theory proposed that two things are happen before emotion occurs. The physical arousal and labeling of the arousal based on cures from the surrounding environment. These two things happen at the same time resulting emotional state. For example, on confronting a wild animal, the physical symptoms (increased heart rate, dilation of pupil and sweating) is accompanied by cognitive (fear of attack or biting) aspects with it. So, at the same time we are able to experience emotion.

MEASUREMENT OF EMOTIONS

It is necessary to learn measurement of the emotions to understand the physiological basis of emotion. Some of the important measurement techniques are explained here.

- **Electroencephalogram (EEG):** EEG measures the changes in brain waves due to emotional arousal. Changes in brain waves are recorded in alternation of different waves.
- **Electrocardiogram (ECG):** ECG record the changes in heart rate due to emotional arousal. For example, changes in various waves due to increased heart rate.
- **Galvanic skin response (GSR):** This test measures the changes skin due to activation of sweat glands.
- **Biofeedback device:** This is another measurement device for measuring changes in various bodily system especially muscle stretching due to emotional arousal.

EMOTION IN HEALTH AND SICKNESS

Emotion and health have direct relation to each others. Changes in emotional state predispose many changes in physical and psychological heath. Long-term emotional disturbance have negative impact on mental as well as on physical health of an individual. For example, long-term sadness may predispose depression and slow down various physiological systems, i.e. loss of appetite, sleep, etc. Emotional changes can also be observed in the form of behavioral problem like severe irritation, frequent aggression, maladjusted family and professional relationship, etc. some of the important emotional disorders are discussed here in brief.

Depression

It is one of the common emotional disorders in world. It is characterized by feelings of sadness, dejection, hopelessness, helplessness and worthlessness. Depression accompanied by many physical and psychological problems like lack of sleep, hunger, slow digestion process, thought of suicide, etc.

Anxiety

Anxiety is also common emotional disorder in individuals. Anxiety is characterized by feelings of apprehension and may predispose to many psychological, physiological and behavioral problems.

Mania

Mania is characterized by excessive talk, speech, loudness of voice, feelings of full of energy and blush. A manic patient might be harmful for self as well as for others.

Implications of Emotions in Nursing

As a nurse, you should concern with your own emotions as well as emotions of patients. Adequate knowledge of emotion and related things will make you much more productive and appreciated at workplace. As a good nurse you should be aware about different emotional reactions, i.e. crying, sadness, shouting, laughing, etc. An adequate and proper knowledge of emotions help a nurse to deal with different kinds of patient in day-to-day life. It will help a nurse in following ways:

- **Understand negative emotions:** Usually sickness changes the emotion state of individual to negative state. Therefore, a nurse should know how to control the negative emotions of the patients.
- **Promote positive emotions:** A well-trained nurse enable a patient to eliminate negative emotions such as anger, fear, worry, and resentment to positive emotions like happiness and joy.
- **Control stress in life:** Proper use of sense of humor and coping strategies will helps to control the stress and its consequences on physical as well as mental health. For example, listening music, going exercise daily, dancing and playing games are positive coping strategies.
- **Prevention of psychosomatic illness:** Improper handling of emotions predisposes many psychosomatic illnesses, i.e.

chronic stress lead to many physical problem, i.e. heart disease, diabetes mellitus, peptic ulcer and psychological disorders, i.e. depression and aggression.

- **Balance in different sphere of life:** Win over emotion help to maintain a balance in different domain of life, i.e. family, home, and neighbor and profession. Failure to win over emotional problems leads to disorganization in personal and professional life.

Suggested Reading

- Babu S. Psychology for Nurses. New Delhi, Elsevier Publication, 2014.
- Morgan CT, King RA, Weiz JR, et al. Introduction to Psychology, 7th edn. New Delhi. Tata McGraw Hill Publishing Company Ltd, 2007.
- Plotnik R. Introduction to Psychology, 5th edn. USA, Wadsworth Publishing Company, 1999.

REVIEW QUESTIONS

SHORT-ESSAY TYPE QUESTIONS

1. Define motivation and discuss motivation cycle.
2. Discuss Maslow's theory of motivation.
3. Define emotion. Explain theory of emotion.

MULTIPLE CHOICE QUESTIONS

1. Which of the following human needs are grouped on lowest level in need in hierarchy of Abraham Maslow?
   a. Physiological needs b. Psychological needs
   c. Self-actualization d. Safety needs
2. Which one is the primary motive?
   a. Hunger b. Affiliation
   c. Aggression d. Achievement
3. Which of the following is NOT an element of motivational cycle?
   a. Need b. Drive
   c. Perception d. Goal and incentive

4. It is the first primitive emotion develops in newborn and human being.
   a. Laughing
   b. Anger
   c. Crying
   d. Love
5. It is a stage in which two motives are equally attracted in an individual at a time.
   a. Avoidance-avoidance
   b. Approach-approach
   c. Multiple approach-avoidance
   d. Approach-approach
6. According to Herzberg's two-factor theory, which of the following is NOT a hygiene factors?
   a. Salary
   b. Status
   c. Job security
   d. Growth
7. The need to purse of influence other is called:
   a. Power motive
   b. Hunger motive
   c. Social motive
   d. Affiliation motive
8. A tendency to harm or damage to other, either physically or psychologically, is called:
   a. Maternal motive
   b. Power motive
   c. Achievement motive
   d. Aggression motive
9. Instinct always oriented to seek pleasure and satisfaction is come under the category of:
   a. Life instincts
   b. Death instincts
   c. Social instincts
   d. Cultural instincts
10. Which of the following is an example of goal directed behavior?
    a. Emotion
    b. Motivation
    c. Tension
    d. Conflict
11. According to which theory emotional changes are the results of visceral and motor reactions in the bodily system and these changes are interpreted in term of emotional feelings.
    a. Canon-Bard theory
    b. James-Lange theory
    c. Schachter-Singer theory
    d. Roger's theory

ANSWER KEY

1.	a	2.	a	3.	c	4.	c	5.	b	6.	d	7.	a
8.	d	9.	a	10.	b	11.	b						

Chapter 9

Stress, Conflict and Frustration

Example 1

Mr Ayush 32-year-old male from a middle class family was staying with his parents, younger sister and a brother. Both parents were retired and younger siblings were studying. He was working in a multinational company as an administrator from last 2 years. He was promoted and was assigned with several responsibilities at work. He got married at the same time he was promoted, thereafter he started having difficulty in completing his tasks at home and office, he started getting tensed and tired too quickly. At the same time his boss gave him an opportunity to work in USA for period of 2 years. He was in dilemma about to continue his job and stay at home or accept the opportunity given by his boss and move to USA for 2 years. Due to his financial status and household responsibilities he was unable to go to USA. Later he regretted for not going to USA and started feeling guilty about his own decision and lost his self-confidence, his work productivity was reduced. What can help him to overcome this?

INTRODUCTION

Stress is a natural human response to day-to-day pressure/ changes experienced by an individual. The term stress has many definitions (Lazarus and Folkman, 1984). Stress is a natural human response to pressure when faced with challenging and sometimes dangerous situations. That pressure is not only about what is happening around us, but often also about demands we place on ourselves. Experiencing stress is part of being alive and some stress helps increase our alertness and energy to meet challenging situations. At certain level stress-helps a person to improve his efficiency at work. If it exceeds beyond ones tolerance level it may lead to poor coping and other stress-related health problems.

If stress lasts for a long time or overwhelms our ability to cope, it can have negative effects on our health, wellbeing, relationships, work and general enjoyment of life. Stress does not have to control our lives. We can improve our knowledge about stress and increase our resources to become more resilient.

DEFINITION

'Stress is the nonspecific response of the body to any kind of demand made upon it.' (Hans Selye,1956)

'Stress is a process in which environmental demands tax or exceeds the adaptive capacity of an organism, resulting in psychological and biological changes that may place persons at risk for disease. (Kessler and Gordon, 1995)

'Stress refers to an imbalance between a perceived demand and the perceived ability of the individual to respond to it.' (McGrath, 1970)

'Stress is the arousal of mind and body in response to demands made upon them.' (Schafer, 2000)

In the above example Mr Ayush when he was exposed to too many responsibilities from his work as well as his personal life hence he had stress which was evident through fatigue, increased tension and difficulty in completing the task in hand.

Theories of stress assume that there is:

- A stressor that poses a demand, challenge or threat
- An awareness or perception of the stressor
- A response that includes emotional, cognitive, behavioral and physiological changes.

Some times when person do not understand how to respond and reacts under stressful situation but frequent exposure to stressful situation makes them familiar to respond in different stressful situation.

Example 2

Usha was studying in first year BSc nursing, while writing nursing care plan she committed several mistakes. Repeatedly she got scolding from her teacher for not writing it well. She started getting tensed while writing it and was finding it difficult to perform good enough in practical and clinical areas. One day she meets her senior who had similar experience during her first year. She listened to her problems, encouraged to write it and gave a few tips to write the care plan. Now Usha is in her final year and she is able to write nursing care plan for any patient she gets in any circumstances. She also started guiding her junior students to improve their skills.

Stress can act as a turning point for better or for worse in a person's life. Once stressors cross person's tolerance/productivity level it start giving unpleasant feeling to person known as distress. Production of distress may vary from person-to-person. But many stressors are very common to majority of people.

In Mr Ayush's case he could not cope with the demands and experienced stress which worsened his life whereas in Usha's case she learned to overcome it and achieved mastery in the area which was stressful to her once.

TYPES OF STRESSOR

Any stimulus which leads to stress can be termed as stressor. These stressors can be divided into two main categories based on the source of the stress — i. intrinsic stressor and ii. extrinsic stressor. Intrinsic stressors are the stressors which are present within an individual; they can also be called as intrapersonal stressors. Extrinsic stressors are the stressors present in person's surrounding; it can be interpersonal, environmental, social stressors. Stressors can also be classified based on duration acute time limited, chronic intermittent, chronic enduring stressors.

- **Intrapersonal stressors:** These stressors are present within an individual such as person's perception, attitude, low tolerance, poor coping skills, inability to perform own duties, pregnancy, sexual difficulty, health problems, changes in daily routine, retirement, unmet physical/psychological/social needs, personal habits, etc.
- **Interpersonal stressors:** These stressors are present between two or more people such as poor communication, strained interpersonal relationship, important life events such as marriage, getting a new family member, divorce, death of near ones, undue expectations by people around, arguments, daily hassles, fights, etc.
- **Environmental stressors:** These stressors are present in surrounding environment such as climatic changes, hospitalization, change in school, new job, catastrophic environment, disasters, etc.
- **Social stressors:** These stressors are present in the society where person resides which includes social status, social isolation, examinations, social events, concerns about standards, responsibilities, acceptance, changes in financial status, social stigma, sociocultural practices, etc.

RESPONSE OF BODY TO STRESSORS

Human body is a complex structure which responds to internal and external stimuli in its own ways. The stimuli experienced by body may come in different forms such as physical/ physiological, psychological, social stimuli. Whenever it extends beyond body's capacity to handle it generates certain amount of stress and body responds to it by physiological, psychological and social response as discussed further.

- **Physiological response:** Various neuroendocrinal mechanisms which are explained in general adaptation syndrome (GAS). Autonomic nervous system responds through sympathetic and parasympathetic response, i.e. fight or flight response. Can be seen overtly by increased mental activity, dilated pupils, bronchial dilatation, increased respiratory rate, increased heart rate, increased glucose, increased cardiac output, increased blood pressure, increased blood flow to the skeletal muscles.
- **Psychological response:** By using various defense mechanisms as discussed under coping mechanisms to maintain the internal harmony of self.
- **Social response:** Seeking social approval, social support for ventilation and distraction from stress provoking situation can enhance the coping of individual.

  Body responds to these intrinsic and extrinsic stressors quickly by fight or flight mechanism. This concept explained very well by stress model, general adaptation syndrome (GAS).

SOURCES OF STRESS

Stress can be caused by several sources such as intrinsic sources (intrapersonal) and extrinsic sources (interpersonal, environmental, social stressors).

- **Intrapersonal sources:** These sources are present within an individual such as person's perception, attitude, personal inadequacies, low tolerance, poor coping skills, inability to perform own duties, pregnancy, sexual difficulty, health problems, changes in daily routine, retirement, unmet physical/ psychological/social needs, personal habits, hereditary illness, attitude towards any illness, and personality traits, etc.
- **Interpersonal sources:** It includes life's daily hassles, inability to adjust with individual differences, adjustments. These

sources are present between two or more people such as poor communication, strained interpersonal relationship, important life events such as marriage, getting a new family member, divorce, death of near ones, undue expectations by people around, arguments, daily hassles, fights, etc.

- **Environmental sources:** It includes catastrophic life events. These sources are present in surrounding environment such as climatic changes, hospitalization, change in school, new job, catastrophic environment, and disasters, etc.
- **Society related sources:** Social status, social discrimination (on account of age, sex, religion, caste, etc.), social isolation, poor social support, examinations, social events, concerns about standards, responsibilities, acceptance, changes in financial status, social stigma, and sociocultural practices, etc.

MODELS OF STRESS

Models of stress assist nurses to identify the stressors. It helps the nurse to predict individual response. Nurse can use this model to assist patient in strengthening healthy coping and in adjusting unhealthy response. There are many models of stress, and only response-based model is discussed here.

- Response-based model: General adaptation syndrome (GAS)
- Transactional model of stress and coping
- Effort-reward imbalance
- The job characteristics model
- The vitamin model.

Response-based Model: GAS

Stress may be considered as response. According to Selye, stress response is characterized by a chain or pattern of physiological events called GAS. The GAS is physiological response of the body towards stress. It is collective response of autonomic nervous system and the endocrine system.

General Adaptation Syndrome (GAS)

Hans Selye (1956–76) has termed the body's response to stressors as the general adaptation syndrome. The general adaptation syndrome consists of three stages: i. alarm reaction, ii. the stage of resistance, and iii. the stage of exhaustion (Fig. 9.1).

Alarm Reaction

It is an emergency response of the body to stressor usually it is mediated by sympathetic nervous system; it prepares us to cope with the stressors.

The Stage of Resistance

If stressors persists the resistance stage begins. During this stage, body starts to defend the stressors by releasing certain hormones such as adrenocorticotropic hormone (ACTH), cortisol and other similar hormones which allow body to deal adaptively with stressors for long period of time. But high levels of these may have harmful effect such as increased blood sugar level by glycogenolysis, impairment in body's immune function by reducing proteins. Several minute changes may occur due to high levels of these hormones, major described here.

The Stage of Exhaustion

The final stage of GAS, here body gets exhausted to the continuous stressors and body's capacity to respond gets seriously compromised.

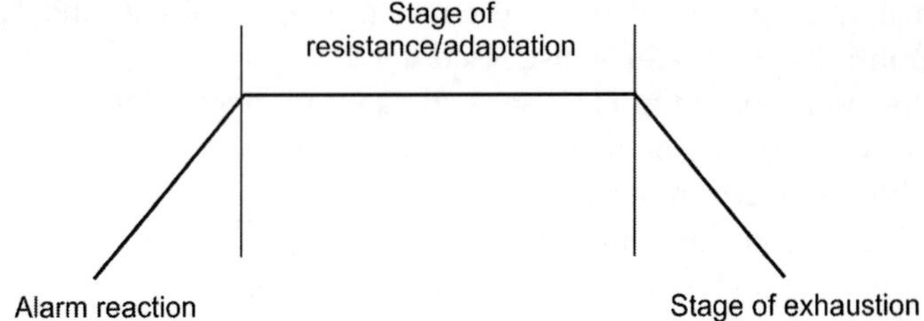

Fig. 9.1: General adaptation syndrome (GAS)

SYMPTOMS OF STRESS

The symptoms of stress can be enumerated under following two headings.

Psychological indicators	Physical and behavioral indicator
Inability to concentrate	Headache
Poor judgment	Muscle tension
Racing thoughts	Nausea
Moodiness	Insomnia

Contd...

Contd...

Agitation	Acne breakout
Irritability	Diarrhea
Loneliness	Loss of sex drive
Constant worrying	Frequently being sick
Negativity	Dizziness
Restlessness	Weight gain
Quick temper	Change in appetite
Sense of being overwhelmed	Neglect
Unhappiness	Drug use
Fearful	Nail biting
Anxiousness	Excessive spending
Indecisiveness	Tooth grinding
Inability to relax	Excessive exercise
Feeling on edge	Overreaction
	Sleeping to much or little
	Starting fight

STRESS ADAPTATION—COPING STRATEGIES

Body has its own mechanism for protection and maintenance of internal harmony. For example, any object coming towards body in a force we close our eyes or try to resist by our extremities or in case we get infected by any bacteria our immune systems starts functioning by increasing the white blood cells which can fight against that infectious microorganism.

Similarly, while person is undergoing stress for protecting oneself against these psychological dangers or distress we use devices such as mental mechanisms or called as defence mechanisms which will help us to protect against any distressing situations. These mental mechanisms help to reduce distress caused by frustration and conflicts. These mechanisms include primary, psychotic/narcissistic, neurotic/immature and mature defence mechanisms.

No ego defence mechanism is psychotic, neurotic, immature, mature or normal *per se*. Almost all mechanisms of defence are sometimes used in normal individuals. Exclusive or abnormally excessive use of a particular defence mechanism makes a defence mechanism neurotic or psychotic.

Defence mechanisms are classified under following broad headings:

Primary Defence Mechanisms

Repression: Unconsciously excluding from conscious awareness of anxiety provoking ideas and/or feelings. For example, forgetting and slips of the tongue.

Psychotic/Narcissistic Defence Mechanisms

- **Regression:** Reversion to modes of psychological functioning that are characteristic of earlier life stages, especially childhood years. For example, dreams, regression in the service of ego (ability of a mature adult to appropriately indulge periodically in playful child-like activities).
- **Denial:** Involuntary exclusion of unpleasant or painful reality from conscious awareness. Commonly seen in grief, and children (3–6-year-old).
- **Projection:** Unconscious attribution of one's own attitudes and urges to other person(s), because of intolerance or painful affect aroused by those attitudes and urges. A universal phenomenon though occurs more commonly in children, persecutory delusions and hallucinations.
- **Distortion:** Unconscious gross 'reshaping' of external reality to satisfy inner needs. Commonly seen in hallucinations, delusions, especially of grandiosity.

Neurotic/Immature Defence Mechanism

- **Conversion:** A repressed, forbidden urge is simultaneously kept out of awareness and also expressed in symbolic/disguised form of some somatic conversion 'reaction' (usually either motor or sensory). Sometimes seen in normal individuals when exposed to catastrophic stress; otherwise presence always implies.
- **Dissociation:** Involuntary splitting or suppression of a mental function or a group of mental functions from rest of the personality in a manner that allows expression of forbidden unconscious impulses without having any sense of responsibility for actions. Near death experience is a example of dissociative disorders.
- **Displacement:** Unconscious shifting of emotions, usually aroused by perceived threat, from an unconscious impulse to

a less threatening external object which is then felt to be the source of threat normal, day-to-day deflection of 'anger' on a substitute target.

- **Isolation (isolation of affect):** Separation of the idea of an unconscious impulse from its appropriate affect, thus allowing only the idea and not the associated affect to enter awareness, e.g. grief, ability to discuss traumatic events without the associated disturbing emotions, with passage of time obsessional thoughts.
- **Reaction formation:** Unconscious transformation of unacceptable impulses into exactly opposite attitudes, impulses, feelings or behaviors. Normal character formation in childhood (from 3 years onwards).
- **Undoing:** Unconsciously motivated acts which magically/ symbolically counteract unacceptable thoughts, impulses or acts, e.g. checking of gas knobs or locks to ensure safety, automatically saying 'I am sorry' on bumping into somebody.
- **Rationalization:** Providing 'logical' explanations for irrational behavior motivated by unacceptable unconscious wishes. A universal phenomenon usually used to explain behaviors, resulting from other defence mechanisms.
- **Intellectualization:** Excessive use of intellectual processes (logic) to avoid affective expression (emotion). When faced with stressful situation, use of logic to focus closely on external reality and avoiding expression of inner feelings (e.g. fear).
- **Acting out:** Expression of an unconscious impulse, through action, thereby gratifying the impulse. Destruction of any object in 'fit of rage'.
- **Schizoid fantasy:** Withdrawal into self to gratify frustrated wishes by fantasy, e.g. seen in adolescence (wish fulfilling daydreams).
- **Turning against thyself (retroflexion):** Unconscious deflection of hostility towards another person onto oneself resulting in lowered self-esteem, self-criticism and at times injury to self, e.g. head banging in children, destruction of property or self in a fit of rage, suicide.
- **Introjection:** Unconscious internalization of the qualities of an objector person. For example, identification with the aggressor (e.g. sometimes seen in victims kidnapped by terrorists; also known as Stockholm syndrome, and grief reaction).

- **Hypochondriasis:** Unconscious transformation of unacceptable impulses into inappropriate somatic concern. Abnormal illness behavior in physically disordered or normal individuals.
- **Inhibition:** Involuntary decrease or loss of motivation to engage in some goal-directed activity to prevents anxiety arising out of conflicts with unacceptable impulses, e.g. writing 'blocks' or work 'blocks', social shyness.
- **Compensation:** (Counter-phobic defence). Unconscious tendency to deal with a fear or conflict by unusual degree of effort in the opposite direction. For example, involvement in dare-devil activities (e.g. sky diving to counter fear of heights), excessive preoccupation with body building to counter feelings of inferiority.
- **Splitting:** Unconscious viewing of self or others as either good or bad without considering the whole range of qualities. Believing personalities to be either 'black' or 'white 'without the shades of 'grey'(e.g. in a 'typical' bollywood movie, the hero often is all good and the villain all bad).

Mature Defence Mechanism

- **Sublimation:** Unconscious gradual channelization of unacceptable infantile impulses into personally satisfying and socially valuable behavior patterns. For example, channelization of sexual or aggressive impulses into creative activities (e.g. diverting forbidden sexual impulses into artistic paintings).
- **Suppression (voluntary):** Voluntary postponement of focusing of attention on an impulse which has reached conscious awareness. For example, voluntary decision not to think about an argument with a close friend while going for an interview.
- **Anticipation:** Realistic thinking and planning about future unpleasurable events. For example, anticipation is a universal phenomenon occurring in all intelligent individuals.
- **Humor:** Overt expression of unacceptable impulses using humor in a manner which does not produce unpleasantness in self or others. It is a universal phenomenon.

STRESS MANAGEMENT

Stress and its responses needs to be addressed appropriately in order to maintain homeostasis and psychological wellbeing.

Prolonged stress may lead to physical problem such as peptic ulcers and other stress-related psychological problems such as generalize/ specific anxiety disorders, phobia, posttraumatic stress disorders, dissociative/somatoform disorders altogether can be called as neurotic or stress-related disorders. Following are the ways which can help in management of stress.

Improving Psychological Response/ Strengthening Coping Mechanisms

The way person responds to stress can be improved by teaching various coping skills, with practice person learns it and handles stressful situation in an effective way without causing any physical or psychological problems to self and others.

- It is also referred to coping mechanism
- The most important nursing intervention is to enhance the coping mechanism of the disease person
- Mccloskey and Bulechek (1999) identifies 'coping enhancement' as a nursing intervention and defined it as 'assisting a patient to adapt to perceive stressors, changes or threats that interfere with meeting demands and rules
- Trying to be optimistic about the outcome
- Using social support
- Using spiritual resources
- Trying to accept the situation
- Trying to maintain control over the feelings.

Promoting Healthy Lifestyle

Healthy lifestyle can influence person's perception about stressors and thereby help them to overcome it by engaging in productive work, defocusing from stressors and using a way of coping by enhancing other skills and capabilities.

- Go for regular exercise
- Take adequate rest and sleep
- Take a well-balanced and nutritious diet
- Adopt positive lifestyle
- Stop smoking, and alcohol ingestion
- Time management
- Do meditation and yoga daily.

Teaching Relaxation Techniques

Use of various relaxation techniques does help in diversion as well as physical and mental relaxation.

- Calm and quiet environment
- Comfortable position
- Passive attitude (over look nature)
- Mental device
- Breathing exercises
- Massage
- Imagery
- Yoga
- Meditation
- Therapeutic touch
- Music therapy
- Laughter therapy.

Strengthen Family Support System

Family has a huge impact on individual's perceptions about the problems and ways of managing stressful situation. A child who witnesses anger and aggression may tend to respond aggressively hence.

- Do the assessment of the family
- Major life events should be explored
- Family coping strategies to be strengthen
- Encourage the family members to stay with person during stressful situations.

Management of Emotional and Behavioral Issues

It involves teaching various skills such as anger control, control of emotional outbursts, etc.

- Individual personality involves a complex relationship among many factors.
- The emotional issues determined by examine the client's current lifestyle, stressors, prior experience with stressors, past successful coping mechanism.

CONFLICT

Conflict is difficult to define, because it occurs in many different settings. The essence of conflict seems to be disagreement, contradiction, or incompatibility. Thus, conflict refers to any situation in which there are incompatible Goals, Cognitions, or Emotions within or between individuals or groups that lead to opposition or antagonistic interaction. Excess conflict may hinder person's ability to take decisions and be focused on tasks and may lead to neurotic disorders if not managed properly. Having self-determination and self-confidence can help an individual to get rid of conflicts.

Definition

Conflict can be defined as opposition between two simultaneous but incompatible feelings. It can also define as a state of opposition between persons or ideas or interests.

Types of Conflict

Conflicts occurring within an individual are basically of four types:

Approach-Approach Conflict

Approach–approach conflict is the simplest form of conflict occurring when two positive goals are equally attractive. The person gets attracted to each but both together are incompatible (Fig. 9.2A). Example: 1) You wanted to see two movies first day first show but both get released on same day. 2) You got selected in renowned international college and same time you get an excellent marriage proposal.

Avoidance-Avoidance Conflict

Conflict occurring when you are forced to select between two negative goals, it takes time to resolve due to persons inability to decide between two threats, fears or situations which are equally not expected by an individual and he tries to avoid it by escaping the situation, freezing or being indecisive (Fig. 9.2B).
Example: Family forcing you to marry against your wish and it is difficult for you to stay at home; you may run away from home or stay away from family and avoid these situations for time being or may not do so thinking about consequences after your action.

Approach-Avoidance Conflict

When person is attracted and repelled by same goal then it becomes very difficult to resolve such conflict (Fig. 9.2C).
Example: A person who is getting emotionally abused by partner but still love each other. It is difficult to decide to terminate the relationship or stay together.

Multiple Approach-Avoidance Conflict

Many of life's problems involve many positive and many negative goals (Fig. 9.2D). Such multiple approach-avoidance conflict does consume a lot of energy of an individual to overcome it. Person may try to use variety of styles of thinking and defence mechanism to overcome it. This conflict may look mixture of all other types of conflicts.

Example: A girl who wants to marry and make her career in her work simultaneously. While working she gets good promotion opportunities as well as good marriage proposals but she is unable to choose the exact one among all which will fulfill her all expectations.

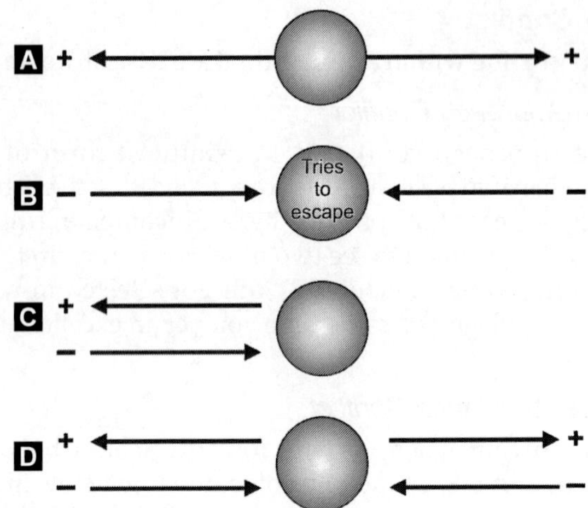

Figs 9.2A to D: Types of conflict: **A.** Approach-approach conflict; **B.** Avoidance-avoidance conflict; **C.** Approach-avoidance conflict; **D.** Multiple approach-avoidance conflict

Levels of Conflict

There can be five levels of conflict such as: i. intrapersonal (within an individual), ii. interpersonal (between individuals), iii. intragroup (within a group), iv. intergroup (between groups), and v. intraorganizational (within organizations).

- **Intrapersonal (within an individual) conflict:** In intrapersonal conflicts there are multiple positive or negative goals or life situations occur at a time in an individual. Approach-approach and multiple approach-avoidance conflicts are few examples of intrapersonal conflicts.

- **Interpersonal (between individuals) conflict:** Interpersonal conflict occurs between two or more than two individuals. Example: two school teachers competing for the same promotion.
- **Intragroup (within a group) conflict:** Conflict can arise in a group because of not matching thinking and understanding level for a particular decision or thing. A group experiencing intragroup conflict may eventually resolve it, allowing the group to reach a consensus. Or the group may not resolve the conflict, and the group discussion may end in disagreement among the members.
- **Intergroup (between groups) conflict:** An organization is a collection of individuals and groups. As the situation and requirements demand, the individuals form various groups. The success of the organization as a whole depends upon the harmonial relations among all interdependent groups, even though some intergroup conflicts in organizations are inevitable.
- **Intraorganizational conflict:** It arises in between an organization while working with different kind of workers. Intraorganizational conflict could be: (i) vertical conflict, (ii) horizontal conflict, (iii) line-staff conflict and (iv) role conflict. Although these types of conflict can overlap, especially with role conflict, each has distinctive characteristics.
    1. **Vertical conflict:** Vertical conflict refers to any conflict between levels in an organization; superior-subordinate conflict is one example. Vertical conflicts usually arise because superiors attempt to control subordinates.
    2. **Horizontal conflict:** Horizontal conflict occurs between employees or departments as the same hierarchical level in an organization.
    3. **Line-staff conflict:** Most organizations have staff departments to assist the line departments. The line-staff relationship frequently involves conflict. Staff managers and line managers typically have different personal characteristics. Staff employees tend to have a higher level of education, come from different backgrounds, and are younger than line employees. These different personal characteristics are frequently associated with different values and beliefs, and the surfacing of these different values tends to create conflict.

4. **Role conflict:** A role is the cluster of activities that others expect individuals to perform in their position. A role frequently involves conflict.

Causes of Conflict

Intrapersonal Causes

Intrapersonal conflict is very common and it may occur due to own perception about the goals, self-confidence, self-respect, knowledge about own capability and weakness, ability to solve own problems using variety of techniques or coping mechanisms.

Individual Differences

No two men are alike in their nature, attitudes, ideals and interests. On account of these differences they fail to accommodate themselves which may lead to conflict among them.

Cultural Differences

Culture is the way of life of a group. The culture of a group differs from the culture of the other groups. The cultural differences among the groups sometimes cause tension and lead to conflict. The religious differences have occasionally led to wars and persecution in history. India was partitioned in the name of religious differences.

Clash of Interests

The interests of different people or groups occasionally clash. Thus the interests of the workers clash with those of the employers which leads to conflict among them.

Social Change

Social change becomes a cause of conflict when a part of society does net change along with changes in the other parts. Social change causes cultural lag which leads to conflict. The parent-youth conflict is the result of social change. In short, conflict is an expression of social disequilibrium.

Conflict Resolution and Techniques

Conflicts resolution depends upon the type of conflict.

- The double approach conflict may be easily resolved by satisfying first one goal which is more important than the other; for instance, a student attending the class first, then going for food even if hungry. Alternatively, this conflict is resolved by giving up one of the goals. Obviously, approach-approach conflict does not generate much anxiety, because the individual is not going to lose much.

- The double avoidance conflict is more complex. Since the individual does not want either of the goals, he experiences more repelling effect as he moves near one goal by rejecting the other. Finally when it is unbearable, the individual tries to leave the conflict situation, but the other factors in periphery of the situation makes it difficult.
- In approach-avoidance conflict, since there is only one goal object, it is very difficult to decide. Here, compromise with the situation is the only alternative solution to overcome stress resulting from conflict.
- Finally, in multiple approach-avoidance conflict the individual has to take a decision depending upon the sum total of positive or negative valences resulting in selection of goals.
- Though these are the coping strategies at individual level, people facing conflicts may help themselves by examining the causes of conflicts clearly, trying to choose the best alternative, early decision making, etc.
- They have to make use of their creative thinking, divergent reasoning and proper perception of the situations.
- Motives may influence our behavior, but the individual should not be the slave of his motives, instead he should be the master of his motives, so that he can have control over them.
- Finally taking advice from parents, elders, teachers and counsellors will be of great help to cope with and to resolve conflicts.

FRUSTRATION

Frustration is a condition of extreme tension, it is commonly interpreted as strong emotional tension caused by blocking of impulses. A person is said to be frustrated because he does not know how to rid himself of his tensions and is therefore highly uncomfortable.

Causes of Frustration

The causes or sources of frustration are found in environmental factors that block motive fulfilment, personal inadequacies that make it impossible to reach goals, and conflicts between and among motives.

- **Environmental factors that block motive fulfilment:** It affects by making it difficult or impossible for a person to attain a goal, environmental obstacles can frustrate the satisfaction of motives. An obstacle may come in different forms such as physical: you are stuck in a traffic, people: parents insisting you to join one course which you do not want to do, friends and other people around coming in the way of achieving your goal.
- **Personal inadequacies that make it impossible to reach goals:** Unattainable goals are important source of frustration. Parents might expect child to be topper in academics and child also struggles for the same but unable to meet the expectation gives rise to frustration.
- **Conflicts between and among motives:** Major sources of conflict are seen here, in this expression of one motive interferes with expression of other motives. For example, expression of love and social approval or aggression and social approval.

Reactions to Frustration

Existence of frustration may lead to development of various reactions to it. These reactions may come in different forms such as:

- **Simple reactions:** a) increasing the efforts to reduce the cause of frustration after thoroughly assessing it. b) *Compromising:* when repeated trials to reduce frustration becomes ineffective person may try to change the goal or minimize the goal to achieve the sense of achievement. c) *Submissiveness:* at the highest degree of frustration as per individual, he may surrender himself and accept the defeat as inevitable.
- **Violent reactions:** In addition to simple reactions, the individual may become emotionally tense and aggressive. This aggression can be of two types: i. *External aggression* which is directed towards others and ii. *Internal aggression* which is directed towards self.
- Loss of confidence and self-esteem after giving up or not fulfilling the desirable goal which in later period may lead to depression.
- **Task-oriented reaction pattern:** Task-oriented reaction involves making necessary changes in the task/ oneself to reduce the frustration. For example, changing the job/project/ method of work if high levels of frustration. All reaction in this may happen with same phenomenon of attack, withdrawal or compromise as discussed earlier.

- **Adjustment mechanisms:** Person learns to adjust to different habits and people to satisfy own motives.

Management of Frustration

Frustration and conflict may causes stress in an individual which can be managed by:

- Identifying the source of frustration/review the situation: can you change or control it? If you can then proceed with it? If you cannot, then learn to accept it
- Change/modify or use a substitute the goals if required to maintain internal harmony
- Focus one problem at a time
- Strengthen coping mechanisms, identifying personal strength and weaknesses and focusing on positive thinking by focusing on what are the benefits or advantages of your compromised situations/decisions.
- Carefully decide about all important decision, seek opinion of others who understands you and your situation better and in a helpful manner
- Do not hesitate to seek reliable help, e.g. friends, teachers counselors, etc.
- Stick to your decision once taken and forget about the other choices unless you are clearly in the wrong.

Nursing Implications

Nurses who are directly in touch with several patients or persons in hospital, community, and workplace may come across these issues very frequently. A thorough knowledge about this can enhance the productivity. Nursing implications can be described in four: i. nursing practice, ii. nursing education, iii. nursing research and iv. nursing administration.

- **Nursing practice:** This knowledge can help
  - To gain insight into themselves and understand human behavior in detail
  - To understand why do different people react in different ways and way to manage it effectively without hurting anybody in process
  - Improve communication with patient and other health team members for effective patient care
  - To improve the quality of nursing services provided in different scenarios.

- **Nursing education:** This knowledge can help nurse educators
  - To understand student's as well as teacher's psychology while working with them
  - To help student in strengthening their own coping mechanism
  - To teach them effective way to manage these problems for themselves and for others
  - To enhance teaching and learning process
  - To impart quality and value based education to the pupil
  - To demonstrate effective ways to handle these problems.
- **Nursing research:** This knowledge can help
  - To conduct researches on human behaviors in different situations, its implications to variety of fields and society.
- **Nursing administration:** This knowledge can help nurse administrators
  - To understand the subordinates in a better way
  - To develop way to manage such problems if it arises in institution
  - To develop certain policies to manage these problems effectively
  - To reinforce subordinates as and when necessary.

Suggested Reading

- Ahuja N. A Short Textbook of Psychiatry, 6th ed. New Delhi: Jaypee Brothers Medical Publishers (P) Ltd., 2006.
- Anthikad J. Psychology for Graduate Nurses, 4th ed. New Delhi: Jaypee Brothers Medical Publishers (P) Ltd., 2008.
- Benjamin S, Virginia S. Kaplan and Sadock's Synopsis of Psychiatry: Behavioral Sciences/Clinical Psychiatry, 10th ed. Philadelphia: Lippincott Williams & Wilkins, 2007.
- Bhatia BD, Craig M. Elements of Psychology and Mental Health, 1st ed. Hyderabad: Orient Longman, 2006.
- Lazarus RS, Folkman S. Stress Appraisal and Coping, 1st ed. New York: Springer, 1984.
- Morgan CT, King RA, Weiz JR, Schopler J. Introduction to Psychology, 7th ed. New Delhi: Tata McGraw Hill Publishing Company Ltd., 2007.
- Plotnik R. Introduction to Psychology, 5th ed. USA: Wadsworth Publishing Company, 1998.

- Satcher. Mental health: a report of surgeon general. Children and mental health. Washington DC: US; Public Health Services, 2000; 124-219.
- Selye H. The Stress of Life, 1st ed (Rev.). New York: McGraw Hill, 1956.

REVIEW QUESTIONS

SHORT-ESSAY TYPE QUESTIONS

1. Define stress and discuss the general adaption syndrome.
2. Discuss different types of stressors.
3. Discuss the management of stress.
4. Define conflicts and types of conflicts.

MULTIPLE CHOICE QUESTIONS

1. Which of the following is a symptom of stress reaction?
   a. Anxiety b. Perception
   c. Attitude d. Affection
2. General adaption stress model was proposed by:
   a. Cannon-Bard b. James-Lange
   c. Hans Seyle d. Weber Wood
3. Which of the following is a negative coping styles?
   a. Going for a walk b. Taking balanced diet
   c. Listening music d. Road rage
4. Involuntary exclusion of unpleasant or painful reality from conscious awareness is which type of defence mechanism?
   a. Undoing b. Reaction formation
   c. Denial d. Projection
5. Unconscious shifting of emotions usually aroused by perceived threat from an unconscious impulse to a less threatening external object which is then felt to be the source of threat normal is which type of defence mechanism?
   a. Dissociation b. Displacement
   c. Compensation d. Regression

6. It is a type of conflict arise when an individual face two negative situations at the same time.
   a. Avoidance-avoidance
   b. Approach-approach
   c. Approach-avoidance
   d. Multiple approach-avoidance conflict
7. It is a type of conflict arises between two or more than two people.
   a. Interpersonal
   b. Intrapersonal
   c. Intragroup
   d. Intergroup
8. Unconscious transformation of unacceptable impulses into exactly opposite attitudes, impulses, feelings or behavior is an example of ....defence mechanism.
   a. Undoing
   b. Reaction formation
   c. Denial
   d. Projection
9. It is universal phenomena in which an individual with the help of unconscious mind usually used to explain behavior resulting from other defence mechanism.
   a. Undoing
   b. Reaction formation
   c. Rationalization
   d. Projection
10. It is a type of defence mechanism in which an individual deliberately do not want to remember painful experiences of his life and voluntary postpone attention to those events.
    a. Displacement
    b. Undoing
    c. Suppression
    d. Repression
11. Tahir often experiences intense feelings of anger and frustration. In order to cope with these feelings he enrolls in a kickboxing class as an outlet for his emotions. Tahir's actions are an example of which type of defence mechanism?
    a. Projection
    b. Displacement
    c. Repression
    d. Sublimation
12. The kind of conflict in which both hopes and fears are associated with the same action is:
    a. Approach-approach conflict
    b. Avoidance-avoidance conflict
    c. Approach-avoidance conflict
    d. Double approach-avoidance conflict

13. A conflict means or implies:
    a. Disorganization of behavior
    b. Incompetence
    c. Incomparability in motives and for goals
    d. Insecurity in feeling
14. With any conflict, the concept of… is attached.
    a. Valency
    b. Force
    c. Need
    d. All of these
15. The most difficult type of conflict to solve is:
    a. Approach-approach
    b. Avoidance-avoidance
    c. Approach-avoidance
    d. I do not know
16. In order to adjust we take help of mental or defence mechanisms. These are:
    a. Socially approved
    b. Socially disapproved
    c. Socially tolerated
    d. a, b, c, are correct

ANSWER KEY

1.	a	2.	c	3.	d	4.	c	5.	b	6.	a	7.	a
8.	b	9.	c	10.	c	11.	d	12.	c	13.	c	14.	a
15.	c	16.	b										

Chapter 10

Attitude

INTRODUCTION

Attitudes are evaluative statements relating to objects, people or events and thus reflect how one feels about something. Attitude is relatively enduring organization of beliefs around an object or situation, predisposing one to respond in preferential manner. In simple form, the combination of knowledge about a thing and forming a tendency to react is an attitude of a person. People's attitude and values have significant impact on their behavior both in organizational and social context. Symbolically attitude can be shown in the following format:

Attitude = Knowledge + Beliefs

MEANING AND DEFINITION

- The term attitude refers to an individual's mental state, which is based on his/her beliefs or value system, emotions, and the tendency to act in a certain way. One's attitude reflects how one thinks, feels, and behaves in a given situation.
- It is a predisposition to react in a persistent and characteristic manner to some situations, ideas, materials, objects or persons.
- It is a predisposition to respond in a positive or negative way to someone or something in one's environment.

'Attitude is a mental and neural state of readiness, organized through experience, exerting a directive or dynamic influence upon the individuals' response related to objects and situations.'

(Alport)

'Attitude is a persistent tendency to feel and behave in a favorable or unfavorable way towards some object, person or idea.' (Reitz)

'Attitude can be defined as a condition of readiness to be motivated.' (Newcomb)

'Attitude is a pattern of behavior, tendencies or anticipatory readiness, predisposition to adapt in social situations, or simply, the attitude is a response to social stimuli that have been conditioned.'

(La Pierre, 2003)

'Attitude can be defined as a tendency or predisposition to evaluate an object or symbol of that in a certain way; evaluation consists of attributing goodness-badness or desirable or undesirable qualities of an object.' (Katz and Scotland)

So, we can conclude that attitude can be defined as our response to people, places, things, or events in life. It can be referred to as a person's viewpoint, mindset, beliefs, etc. our attitude towards people, places, things, or situations determines the choices that we make.

FEATURES OF ATTITUDE

- **Attitude affects behavior:** Attitude affects the behavior of an individual by putting him/her to respond favorable towards a particular object.
- **Attitudes are acquired or learned:** Attitudes are acquired or learned through learning over a period of time. The process of learning attitudes starts right from the childhood and continue throughout the life of the person.
- **Attitudes are invisible:** Attitudes are invisible as they constitute psychological phenomena which cannot be observed directly. They can be observed by observing the behavior of an individual.
- **Attitudes are pervasive:** Attitudes are pervasive that every individual have some kind of attitude towards the object in the environment.
- **Attitudes are the net product of the socialization process:** Attitudes are the net product of the socialization process as they are reflected in the words and deeds of the individual.
- **Attitudes are relatively enduring and persisting:** They are not behavior but only predispositions to act. Attitudes are not directly known but indirectly inferred from behavior.
- **Attitudes are always goal directed:** Attitudes are always goal directed either in a positive or a negative way.

NATURE OF ATTITUDES

- **Attitudes are relatively stable:** Temporary mood states and one time action cannot be considered as an attitude. Once it is formed it has tendency to persist overtime and across situation. However, it does not mean that attitudes do not change. They do change in the light of new experience and information. Family environment also influence attitudes because it inculcate some experience which always remains with us.

- **Attitudes are dispositional:** Dispositional means that attitudes are the characteristics of an individual and people differ in their strength from one another depending upon their socialization and social interactions.
- Attitudes are related to images, thoughts and external objects.
- Attitudes are not innate.

FUNCTIONS OF ATTITUDE

- They provide basis for defining social groups
- Attitude helps to establish our identity
- Attitude guide thinking and behavior
- It plays an important role at the societal level
- Attitudes facilitate selection of facts
- Other functions includes
  - Motivational functions
  - Ego defensive functions
  - The value expressive and self-realizing functions
  - Attitudes guide information processing
  - Attitudes guide behavior.

COMPONENTS OF ATTITUDE

Attitude is composed of three components, which includes:

1. Cognitive component
2. Affective/emotional component
3. Behavioral component.

Basically, the cognitive component is based on the information or knowledge, whereas affective component is based on the feelings. The behavioral component reflects how the attitude affects the way we act or behave.

For instance, in case of a person who is scared of an injection or a needle, the cognitive component might be the fact that an injection would hurt. On the other hand, the affective component would be the feeling that he/she is scared of injection. The behavioral component would be that the person would completely avoid getting an injection or scream at the sight of one. So, an attitude is essentially like an evaluative statement that is either positive or negative depending on the degree of like or dislike for the matter in question.

TYPES OF ATTITUDE

In general, there are three types of attitudes. These are:

Positive Attitude

Individual who have a positive attitude will pay attention to the good, rather than the bad in people, situations, events, etc. they will not consider a mistake or failure as a hurdle, but as an opportunity. They learn from mistakes, and move forward in life.

Their traits are:

- Confidence
- Optimism
- Cheerfulness/happiness
- Sincerity
- Sense of responsibility
- Flexibility
- Determination
- Reliability
- Tolerance
- Willingness to adapt
- Humility
- Diligence.

Negative Attitude

People with a negative attitude ignore the good and pay attention to the bad in people, situations, events, etc. Also, they are likely to complain about changes, rather than adapting to the changing environment. Also, they might blame their failure on others.

Traits are:

- Anger
- Hatred
- Pessimism
- Frustration
- Doubt
- Resentment
- Jealousy
- Inferiority.

Neutral Attitude

People with a neutral attitude do not give enough importance to situations or events. They ignore the problem, leaving it for someone else to solve. Also, they do not feel the need to change. Their traits include:

- Complacence
- Indifference
- Detachment
- Feeling of being disconnected
- Unemotional.

It must be noted that there is a very thin line between personality traits and attitude. While the former are more rigid and permanent, the latter may change with different situations and experiences in life. So, attitudes are learned and experienced.

Attitude can be explicit or implicit. Attitude at an unconscious level that might be unknown to us and is formed involuntarily is referred to as implicit attitude. On the other hand, explicit attitude refers to the attitude at a conscious level. Implicit attitude might be attributed to past experiences or influences.

Daniel Katz classified attitudes into four different groups based on their functions:

1. **Utilitarian:** It provides us with general approach or avoidance tendencies.
2. **Knowledge:** Help people organize and interpret new information.
3. **Ego-defensive:** Attitudes can help people protect their self-esteem.
4. **Value-expressive:** Used to express central values or beliefs.

Utilitarian

People adopt attitudes that are rewarding and that help them avoid punishment. In other words, any attitude that is adopted in a person's own self-interest is considered to serve a utilitarian function.

Knowledge

People need to maintain an organized, meaningful, and stable view of the world. That being said important values and general principles can provide a framework for our knowledge. Attitudes achieve this goal by making things fit together and make sense. Examples:

- I believe that I am a good person
- I believe that good things happen to good people

- Something bad happens to Raj
- So, I believe Raj must not be a good person.

Ego-defensive

This function involves psychoanalytic principles where people use defense mechanisms to protect themselves from psychological harm. Mechanisms include:

- Denial
- Repression
- Projection
- Rationalization.

We are more likely to use the ego-defensive function when we suffer a frustration or misfortune.

Value-expressive

- Serves to express one's central values and self-concept
- Central values tend to establish our identity and gain us social approval thereby showing us who we are, and what we stand for.

An example would concern attitudes toward a controversial political issue.

DEVELOPMENT OF ATTITUDES

Attitudes are not innate but are learned. They are acquired by us. Some of them are built by us by our effort. Others are absorbed by us passively and spontaneously from the social environment into which we are born and in which we grow. Many of our attitudes are the result of reflection and purposeful thinking or the outcome of training and suggestions from others. The attitude formations are considered all those factors from which a learning process takes place.

Attitudes Formation

Among the determinants of attitudes–the individual's wants, information, group affiliations and personality are the main.

- Attitudes develop in the process of want satisfaction
- The attitudes of the individual are shaped by the information to which he is exposed
- The group affiliations of the individual help to determine the formation of his attitudes
- The attitudes of the individual reflect his personality.

Factors in Attitude Development

- **Family as a group:** For attitude formation, family plays an important role. A newly born child learns behavior firstly from his mother and subsequently from other members of the family. This is known as socialization process where he learns and forms attitude also. Family has two important roles. Firstly, the family members have certain characteristics; evaluate criteria, attitudes and values which are shared by all other persons. In early childhood, through socialization we learn and form attitudes of the family members.

  Secondly, family mediates the influence of the large social system on the individual's attitude, values and personality characteristics.
- **Reference groups:** Reference groups serve as important inputs to an individual's learning of his attitudes and awareness of alternative behaviors and lifestyles. This happens also through the process of socialization though all groups with which an individual make contacts have influence on his attitudes, the value and norms of the primary group play a very important role in influencing attitudes, opinions, values and beliefs.
- **Social group:** The social classes have an important influence on individual's behavior and attitude. They have the important task of transmitting cultural behavioral pattern to specific groups and families.
- **Personality factor:** Personality factors are important in attitude formation, because attitudes of the individual usually reflexes in personality. Many personality characteristics themselves are determined by group and social factors. Various studies shows that there is a positive relationship between different personality factors and attitudes.
- **Economic factors:** A person's attitude towards a host of issues such as pleasure, work, marriage, etc. are influenced by economic factors such as his/her economic status in the society, rate of inflation in the economy, government economic policy and the country's economic condition.
- **Psychological factors:** The psychological makeup of a person is made up of his perception, ideas, values, beliefs, informations, etc. It has a crucial role in determining a person's attitude. For example, if a person perceives that generally all superior are exploitive he/she is likely to develop a negative attitude towards his/her supervisors who is in fact not exploitative.

- **Mass media exposure:** As a means of communication, the mass media such as television, radio, has a major influence in shaping people's opinions and beliefs. There is new information on something that provides the foundation for the emergence of new cognitive attitudes towards it. A strong enough suggestive messages that carry information will also form attitudes toward certain things.
- **Personal experience:** In order to be the basis of attitudes, personal experiences have left a strong impression. Therefore, the attitude will be more easily formed when personal experience involves emotional factors. In situations involving emotions, appreciation will be more in-depth experience and longer trace.
- **Forming attitude by balance:** People prefer consistency or harmony in relationship among their cognitions. People develop sentimental relation with all those with whom they have harmonious relationship.

ATTITUDE CHANGE

Attitude change implies that the issue towards which we are unfavorable produces now an attitude of being favorable towards it. Attitude change means a change in the stand of the individual with regard to a problem. It is very difficult to change the attitude once it have been formed and established. But it is necessary to modify the unhealthy or irrational attitudes for learning new and creative things. The attitude once formed differs in their modifiability, their susceptibility to change and modifiability of an attitude depends upon certain characteristics of the pre-existing attitude and upon certain characteristics of the individual.

The technique by which attitude can be changed depends upon three basic factors.

1. Attitude characteristics and modifiability
2. Personality of attitude holder
3. Group affiliation of the attitude holder.

Attitude Characteristics and Modifiability

In understanding attitude change, the analysis of attitude characteristics is an important element. This include:

- **Extremeness:** A commonly accepted principle is that more extreme attitudes have lower susceptibility to change than do less extreme attitude and hence may be expected to be more resistant to change.

- **Multiplexity:** The modifiability of an attitude may be expected to vary with its degree of multiplexity.
- **Consistency:** A consistent attitude system ends to be a stable one. The components mutually support each other. An inconsistent system is in contrast, relatively unstable because of the dissonance among its component and hence may be more easily changed in the direction of increased consistency.
- **Interconnectedness:** The amount and nature of the interconnectedness of an attitude with other attitudes are important in determining how easily the attitude can be modified.
- **Consonance of attitude cluster:** The ease of changing an attitude which is a part of a cluster will vary with the degree to which it is consonant with the other attitudes in the cluster.
- **Strength and number of wants served:** The resistance of an attitude to change depends partly upon the strength and number of the wants served. An attitude based on the strong and multiple wants, therefore will be relatively immune to incongruent change.
- **Centrality of related values:** Many of the attitudes of the individual reflect his values—his conception of what is good or desirable. An attitude that stems from a value that is basic to the individual and strongly supported by his culture will be difficult to move in an incongruent direction.

Personality of Attitude Holder

The personality factors of attitude holder are also important in attitude change in the sense that some persons are more perusable as compared to others. This is so because of personality difference. Persuability is the tendency of a person to accept a persuasive communication. It commonly refers to a response to a direct influence attempt. Several personality factors suggest different types of persuability.

- First is the level of self-esteem of the person. The more inadequate a person feels and the more social inhibition he has, the more likely is he to be pursuable.
- People with a great deal of confidence in their own intellectual ability are not only more resistant to change but more willing to expose themselves to discrepant information.

- **Close mindedness or dogmatism:** It is a form of authoritarianism where there is admiration of those in authority and hatred for those opposed to authority.

Group Affiliation of the Attitude Holder

Individuals often express their attitudes in terms of group. This is more so in the cases of less extreme attitudes.

FACTORS AFFECTING ATTITUDE CHANGE

- **Source of message or communicator:** The message is originated from the credible, trustworthy and expert person to produce change. Communicators, if similar to the target audience, their message will be well taken. For example, product advertised on the TV by a famous film star in a attractive manner.
- **Characteristic of message or communication**:
  - **Suggestions:** The communication should discuss both pro and cons to the point, e.g. doctor prescribing chemotherapy for the cancer patients but not telling the side effects of the drugs.
  - **Making available new information:** People can be provided with new information to change their attitudes.
  - **Using fear:** The use of fear has also been effectively used to change attitudes. However, the degree of fear must be moderate rather than mild or strong.
- **Characteristic of recipient or audience:** Personality characteristics of the audience have been linked with attitude change. Recipient with gullible or suggestive personality will be easily persuaded for the change.

Methods to Change Attitude

Robbins found that persuasive skills were highly effective in improving the attitude of employees. He thinks that management can induce workers to change their attitude by consciously manipulating what it intends to convey to them.

The pervasive skills involve:

- Establishing management credibility
- Using positive tactful tone
- Making clear presentation
- Providing strong evidence to support management position

- Tailoring argument to the workers
- Employing logic
- Using emotional appeals.

Techniques of attitude change:
- By exposing the individual to an external influence
- By interaction
- By group discussion/lecture.

Psychometric Assessment of Attitude

Attitudes are evaluations. There are different methods to measure attitudes. Broadly it can be measured by:
- **Self-report methods:** In this method a questionnaire or a list of statements related to the attitudinal object are given to the respondent. The response format is either fixed, i.e. categories for the response are named such as agree-disagree, like-dislike, favorable-unfavorable, or left open-ended where respondents can use their own words.
- **Attitude scales:** These are most commonly used for the measurement of attitudes as with these scales, a precise measurement is possible. They generally yield a total score indicating the direction and intensity of an individual's attitude towards an object, event or class of stimuli. There are four methods of constructing attitude scales.
  1. Thurstone type scale
  2. Likert type scale
  3. Guttman's scalogram
  4. Osgood's semantic differential type.
- **Voluntary behavior method:** In these the physiological measures are used. Earlier galvanic skin response and size of the pupil of the eye have been used as the indicator of arousal to measure attitude. These have not been very successful as only extremity of attitudes can be measured and that too the direction of attitude cannot be specified. Recently electromyography recordings from the major facial muscles have been used to measure attitudes, but this has not been successfully established.

Importance of Attitudes in Nursing

The professional attitude of the nurse is not only concerned with her feelings, beliefs and her behavior towards the patients but also towards other elements of professional functioning like health-care delivery, scientific interest and collaboration with other professionals. Importance of study of attitudes for nurses can be related to the following factors:

- **Patient care:** Any negative attitude towards race, community or a disease results in a biased behavior that affects the patients. Many a times stereotypic beliefs, which you might have developed in earlier sociocultural milieu, are not based on rational scientific reasoning. Due to these attitudes you can behave inappropriately. This can interfere with your professional competence.
- **Formation of attitudes of peers or juniors:** Senior nurses have a significant impact on the formation of opinion concerning health-related issues. These attitudes could be learned by other peer nurses, student nurses and other hospital staff associated in the healthcare. One has to be careful that the negative attitudes of one person do not generate similar attitude in the group.
- **Acceptance of new technology:** In the present scenario, many a new innovations in techniques, equipment and methods of healthcare delivery are taking place. Our attitudes can bias our acceptance towards new technology and high profile specialties.
- **Interpersonal skills:** Studies have shown that during the training, there is as gradual decline in the interpersonal skills. This affects history taking, information elicitation from the patient. Studies have also shown that as students increase their clinical experience, their behavior pattern changes.
- **Curriculum planning:** While planning to new curriculum or to revise the existing curriculum in the educational courses one needs to identify the attitudes of students and the teachers. Accordingly attitude change for altered behavior patterns can be seeked and incorporated in the curriculum.
- **Effects of attitudes on meaningful learning and retention:** It is being recognized that besides cognitive factors, positive or negative attitudinal bias has differential effect on the learning of the controversial material. With favorable attitude one is highly motivated to learn, puts greater efforts and concentrates better. Negative attitude leads to close minded view to analyze new material and hence learning is impaired. Attitude structure exerts an additional facilitating influence on recognition and motivation.

Suggested Reading

- Bhatia HR. Textbook of Educational Psychology. Asia Publishing House, 1905; pp 67-78.
- Dwivedi RS. Human Relations and Organizational Behaviour—A Global Perspective, 5th ed, Macmillan Company, 2001; pp 93-8.
- Sreevani R. Psychology for Nurses, 2nd ed. New Delhi: Jaypee Brothers Medical Publishers (P) Ltd. 2013; pp 116-9.
- Stephens JM. Educational Psychology—The Study of Educational Growth, 2nd ed. Henry Holt Company, New York, 1958; pp 531-2.

REVIEW QUESTIONS

SHORT-ESSAY TYPE QUESTIONS

1. Define attitude and explain the process of attitude formation.
2. Discuss different types of attitude.
3. Discuss the factors affecting development of attitude.

MULTIPLE CHOICE QUESTIONS

1. The learned predisposition about something is called:
   a. Attitude   b. Stress
   c. Emotion   d. Anger
2. Which of the following are attitude measurement scales?
   a. Thurstone type scale   b. Likert type scale
   c. Guttman's scalogram   d. All of the above
3. Which of the following component of attitude based on information or knowledge?
   a. Cognitive   b. Affective
   c. Psychomotor   d. None of the above

ANSWER KEY

1.	a	2.	d	3.	a								

Chapter 11

Personality

INTRODUCTION

Why do people behave differently? Do they have a choice to shape their personality the way they want? How do people predict others behaviors? Writers, philosophers have reflected enough thoughts about personality for centuries. They described various types of people.

Number of personality training centers emerged to shape peoples' personality at different levels, to play different roles in the society. Our personality can limit or expand our options and choices in life. It can prevent us from sharing some experiences with certain people and enable us to make one of them

Evidence from a wide range of studies appears to indicate that we are born with unique personalities, but there is still a lot of room for change. Our personalities develop during our early years and continue to change in adulthood in response to age-related and culturally determined demands. But there are also considerable individual differences in the ways that our personalities change in response to life experiences. This suggests that it can be dangerous for healthcare professionals to believe that an individual's personality tells them anything meaningful about the way they are likely to respond to a particular illness or event.

Hence, nurses need to understand how personality evolves across lifespan and the influential factors to shape the personality.

DEFINITION

The word 'personality' originated from the Latin word ***'persona'***, which referred to a Theatrical mask worn by Roman actors in Greek dramas. These ancient Roman actors wore a mask (persona) to project a role or false appearance. Personality is unique, relatively enduring internal and external aspects of a person's character that influence behavior in different situations.

'Personality is the pattern of enduring characteristics that produce consistency and individuality in a given person. It encompasses the behaviors that make each of us unique and that differentiate us from others'.

'Personality refers to deeply ingrained patterns of behavior, which include the way one relates to, perceives and thinks about the environment and oneself'. (APA, 1987)

'Personality refers to an individual's characteristic patterns of thought, emotion and behavior together with the psychological mechanisms hidden or not behind those patterns'.

(Funder, 2004)

'Personality is the organized, developing system within the individual that represents the collective action of that individual's major psychological subsystems'. (Mayer, 2007)

TYPES OF PERSONALITY

Personality type refers to the psychological classification of different kinds of individuals. These are different from personality traits. Personality types explain the qualitative differences between people whereas personality traits might be the quantitative differences. For example, as per type theories—introverts and extroverts are two fundamentally different categories of people.

Some of the commonly used types of personality are discussed here:

- Hippocrates classification of personality
- Kretschmer's classification
- Sheldon's classification
- Jung's classification
- Type A and type B personality.

Hippocrates classification of personality: The Greek physician Hippocrates included four temperaments into medical theories using a concept of humorism that four body fluids affect human personality and behaviors (Table 11.1).

- Sanguine (optimistic and social)
- Phlegmatic (relaxed and peaceful)
- Melancholic (analytical and quiet)
- Choleric (short tempered or irritable).

Table 11.1: Hippocrates classification

Fluid type	Related natural element	Personality type	Characteristics
Blood	Air	Sanguine	Sociable, carefree, talkative, pleasure seeking, talkative, imaginative, artistic, make new friends easily
Phlegm	Water	Phlegmatic	Calm, patient, caring, tolerant, seek a quiet and peaceful atmosphere, consistent with their habits, steady and faithful
Black bile	Earth	Melancholic	Introverted, suspicious, preoccupied with tragedy and cruelty in world, sad, depressive
Yellow bile	Fire	Choleric	Excitable, impulsive, egocentric, restless, passionate

Kretschmer's classification: A German psychiatrist who attempted to correlate body physique and character based on his observations from his patients with mental illness (Table 11.2).

Table 11.2: Kretschmer's classification

Physique type	Characteristics
Pyknic (short, round body)	Extraversion, kind hearted, expressive
Athletic (strong body)	Energetic, aggressive, determined, adventurous and balanced
Asthenic (slender and slim body)	Introverts, sensitive, reserved, pessimistic, not expressive
Dysplastic (unproportionate body)	Imbalanced nature, unpredictable

Sheldon's classification of personality: William Herbert Sheldon explained temperament with human body types (Fig. 11.1 and Table 11.3).

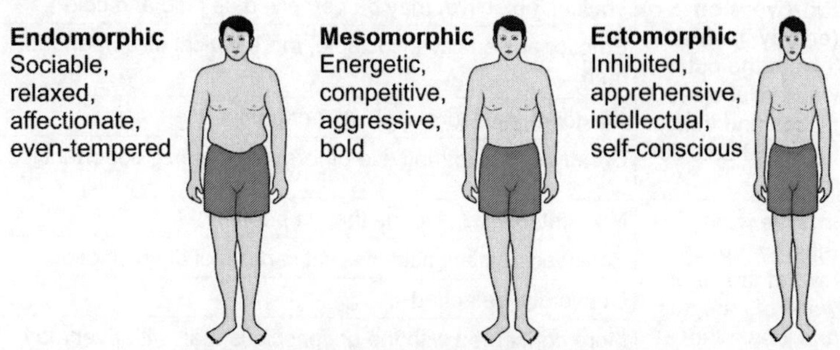

Fig. 11.1: Sheldon's three basic body types

Table 11.3: Sheldon's classification of personality

Sheldon's body type	Shape and description	Characteristics
Endomorphic (viscerotonic)	Plump, highly-developed viscera, but weak somatic structure, i.e. fat, soft and round	Relaxed, sociable, fun-loving, love of food, tolerant, even-tempered, good humored
Mesomorphic (somatotonic)	Muscular, balanced development of viscera and strong somatic structure	Active, assertive, vigorous, loves risk and adventure.
Ectomorphic (cerebrotonic)	Lean and delicate undeveloped viscera and weak somatic structure	Self-conscious, pessimistic, inhibited, introverted, anxious, artistic, emotionally restrained, thoughtful

Jung's classification of personality: Jung divided personality into eight types based on interactions of the attitudes (introversion and extroversion) and the functions (thinking, feeling, sensing and intuiting) (Fig. 11.2 and Table 11.4).

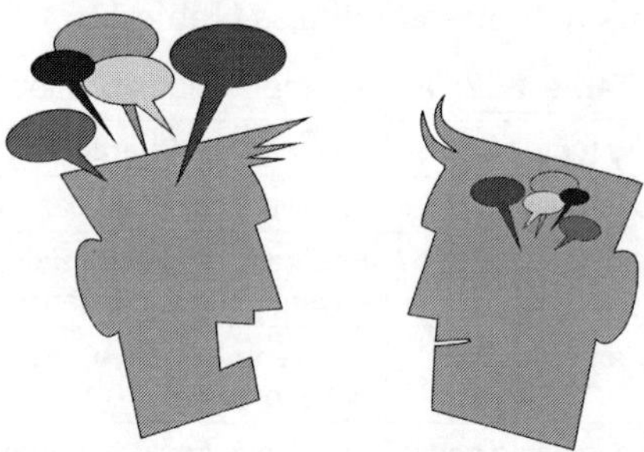

Fig. 11.2: Jung's two basic types of personality

Table 11.4: Jung's classification of personality

Description	Characteristics
Extroversion (energy moves toward the outer world of people, places and things; the world outside of us)	Logical, objective, may be perceived as rigid and cold
	Emotional, sensitive, sociable, more typical of women than men
	Outgoing, pleasure seeking, adaptable
	Creative, able to motivate others and to seize opportunities
Introversion (energy moves toward the inner world of thoughts and ideas; the world inside of us)	More interested in ideas than in people
	Reserved, undemonstrative, yet capable of deep emotion
	Outwardly, detached
	More concerned with the unconscious than with everyday reality

Type A and type B personality (Table 11.5): This typing was first described in relation to heart diseases by cardiologists Meyer Friedman and Rosenman. Type A and B personality are based broadly on anxiety and stress levels which are known to be associated with increased or decreased likelihood of developing coronary artery disease.

Table 11.5: Type A and type B personality

Type A	Type B
• Competitive, outgoing, ambitious, impatient and aggressive • Lives at a higher stress level • They enjoy achievement of goals with greater enjoyment in achieving more difficult goals. They are constantly working hard to achieve • They find difficult to stop, even when have achieved their goals • They live under constant pressure, largely of their own making • They hate failure and difficult to accept failures	• Easy going, relaxed, calm and peaceful • Lives at lower stress levels • They work steadily and enjoying achievements but not becoming stressed when they are not achieved • They can be disappointed but not devastated, they are more of accepting failures • They may be creative enjoy exploring ideas and concepts

FACTORS INFLUENCING PERSONALITY

Personality is a comprehensive concept that emphasizes the growth and behavior of the child as an organized whole. As personality developed within the social framework, there are many factors which contribute to its development. The factors that influence personality can be classified into:

- **Biological factors:** The biological factors are of biogenic by nature and include those of heredity, physique, nervous system, etc.
  - **Heredity:** It refers to physical stature, facial attractiveness, sex, temperament, muscle composition and reflexes are characteristics that are considered to be inherent. Heredity traits are transmitted through genes.
  - **Nervous system:** The architecture of the brain assists in understanding how parts of the brain interact with the reset of nervous system and influence functional expressions, behavior, emotions and personality.
  - **Physique:** It focuses an individual's external appearance which also determines the personality. Physical features

like tall or short, fat or skinny, black or white are physical features which can affect the self-concept of individual.

- **Environmental factors:** The environment of an individual consists of the sum total of the stimulation which he/she receives from conception to birth.
  - **Cultural factors:** Each culture teaches to its members to behave in certain ways that are acceptable to the group. Cultural factors determine an individual's attitudes towards independence, aggression, competition, cooperation, positive thinking, etc.
  - **Family factors:** Family has a major role in developing personality of the children. Birth order, family size and family environment are certain factors which influence the personality.

THEORIES OF PERSONALITY DEVELOPMENT

When discussing any type of development, most theorists break it down into different stages. Developmental theories make out specific behaviors associated with various stages specifying its appropriateness. Nurses should have a basic understanding of human personality development to identify the maladaptive behavioral responses when they deal with patients. The major theoretical approaches of personality include (Table 11.6):

- Psychodynamic approaches to personality
- Lifespan approach
- Trait approaches
- Humanistic approaches
- Behavioral and social learning approaches
- Biological and evolutionary approaches

PSYCHODYNAMIC APPROACHES TO PERSONALITY

The college student wanted to make a good first impression on an attractive girl he had spotted across a crowded room at a party. As he walked toward her, he mulled over a line, he had heard in an old movie the night before: 'I do not believe we have been properly introduced yet.' To his horror, what came out was a bit different. After threading his way through the crowded room, he finally reached the woman and blurted out, 'I do not believe we have been properly seduced yet'.

Table 11.6: Overview of personality theories

Theory	Basic concepts
1. Psychodynamic approaches • Sigmund Freud's psychoanalytic theory • Neo-Freudian psychoanalytical theory – Carl Jung's analytical psychology – Alfred Adler's individual psychology – Karen-Horney psychoanalytic interpersonal theory – Erich Fromm's humanistic psychoanalysis – Henry Murray's theory of personality – Erik Erikson's Psychosocial development	• Emphasizes the unconscious. • Stresses innate, inherited structure of personality while pointing out the importance of childhood experiences • Stresses determinism, the view that behavior is directed and caused by factors outside one's control • Emphasizes the stability of characteristics thought the person's life
2. Trait approaches • Gordon Allport • Raymond Cattell • Hans Eysenck	Disregard conscious and unconscious. Individual's personality is described in an effort to make future behavior
3. Humanistic approaches • Carl Rogers • Abraham Maslow	Focuses on those aspects of personality that make people uniquely human, such as freedom of choice, subjective feelings, etc.
4. Behavioral and social learning approaches • BF Skinner • John Dollard and Neal Miller • Albert Bandura	Focuses on environment, emphasizes the importance of both the influences of other people's behavior and of a person's own expectancies on learning
5. Biological and evolutionary approaches	Focuses on inherited determinants of personality

Although this student's error may seem to be merely an embarrassing slip of the tongue, according to some personality theorists such a mistake is not an error at all. Instead, psychodynamic personality theorists might argue that the error illustrates one way in which behavior is triggered by inner forces that are beyond our awareness. These hidden drives, shaped by childhood experiences, play an important role in energizing and directing everyday behavior.

Psychodynamic approaches to personality are based on the idea that personality is primarily unconscious and motivated by inner forces and conflicts about which people have little awareness. The most important pioneer of the psychodynamic approach was Sigmund Freud. A number of Freud's followers, including Carl

Jung, Karen Horney, and Alfred Adler, refined Freud's theory and developed their own psychodynamic approaches.

- Sigmund Freud's psychoanalytic theory
- Neo-Freudian psychoanalytical theory

Psychoanalytic Theory (Sigmund Freud)

Sigmund Freud who is known as father of Psychiatry, explained about understanding the mapping of mind. He emphasized that the first 5 years of a child's life to be the most important, because individual's basic character had been formed by the age of 5 years.

Freud's personality theory can be explained according to structure and dynamics of the personality, topography of the mind, and stages of personality development.

Topography of the mind/levels of personality (Fig. 11.3): Freud's original perception divided personality into three levels: i. the conscious, ii. the preconscious, and iii. the unconscious.

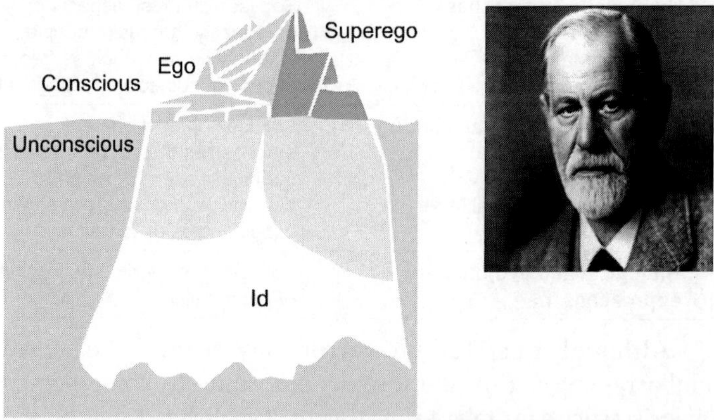

Fig. 11.3: Topography of mind

The conscious: It consists of all the sensations and experiences which we are aware at a given moment. As you read these words for instance; you may be conscious of the feel of your pen, the idea you are trying to get from the passage, moving sound of your fan, etc.

- It is the limited aspect of our personality and only a small portion (around 10%) of our memories, sensations, and thoughts are subject matter of conscious mind.
- Things which are easily remembered or retrieved are considered to be within one's conscious awareness. An individual do not

need to take any sort of efforts to bring back the experience to explain or narrate to others. Examples include telephone numbers, birthdays of self and significant others, dates of special holidays, and what one had for lunch today.

- Freud compared the mind to an iceberg. The conscious is the portion above the surface of water merely the tip of an iceberg.

The unconscious: The larger, invisible portion below the surface of water of an iceberg.

- This is the focus of the psychoanalytic theory.
- Its dark, vast depths are the home of the instincts, those wishes and desires that direct our behavior.
- The unconscious consists of major driving force behind all behaviors which we cannot see or control.
- A major portion (80%) of memories, sensation and thought comes under unconscious portion of the brain. It is almost impossible to bring or retrieve the experience of an individuals' daily experience but use of hypnotism and others ways may helps to bring back the experience.

The preconscious: Between conscious and unconscious level is the preconscious. It only covers 10% of the experiences we have in our daily life.

- It is the storehouse of all memories, perception and thoughts may have been forgotten or are not in present awareness but, with attention, can readily be recalled into consciousness. An individual need little effort to bring the lived experience from subconscious to conscious mind. It is also known as 'tip of tongue phenomena'.
- Examples include telephone numbers or addresses once known but little used and feelings associated with significant life events that may have occurred at some time in the past. In Iceberg theory, a small and floating part is considered preconscious or subconscious part.

Structure of the Personality

Freud organized the structure of the personality into three major components: i. **id**, ii. **ego**, and iii. **superego**. These are abstract conceptions and they do not exist in physical structure of brain. They are different in their unique functions and characteristics (Table 11.7).

- **Id:** It operates on *'pleasure principle'* and present at birth. The id is raw, unorganized and inborn part of the personality and focus on to reduce the immediate tension and maximize the satisfaction. Usually, Id-driven behaviors are impulsive and may be irrational in nature.
- **Ego:** The ego, also called the rational self or the *'reality principle'*. Ego begins to develop soon after the birth; between 4 and 6 months of life. It strives to balance the desires of id and realities of the objective outside the world. Ego is the 'executive' of personality; it makes decisions, controls actions and allows thinking and problem solving. Ego delay the execution of plan of Id. A strong ego will helps to shape and flourish personality of an individual.
- **Superego:** The superego might be referred to as the *'perfection* or *'morality principle'*. It is also known as 'conscience'. Superego is a final personality structure develops in childhood between ages 3 to 6 years which harshly judges the morality of our behavior. It represents the right and wrong of society which is taught and demonstrated by parents, teacher and significant others.
  - Superego formed from rewards and punishments, when a child is consistently rewarded for good behavior his/her self-esteem enhanced. On the contrary, conscience is formed when his/her bad behavior is consistently punished.
  - The superego is essential for socialization of the individual because it assists the ego in the control of id impulses.

Table 11.7: Examples of id, ego and superego

Id	Ego	Superego
'I found this purse; I will keep this money'	'I already have money. This money does not belong to me. May be the person who owns this may not have any money'	'It is never right thing to take something which does not belong to you'
Mom and Dad is not at home. Let me call my friends and enjoy	Mom and dad said no friends when they are away from home. Too risky	Never disobey your parents
In dark lonely night, think to do something wrong with a lonely girl	'No, this is not a right place to do something wrong. Let me wait for a safe place'	'What if she could be my daughter or sister'

Anxiety–A Threat to Ego

Freud described anxiety as an objectless fear very often we cannot point out its source to a specific object or situation which caused the fear. Freud emphasized anxiety as an important part of his personality theory, the reason behind the neurotic and psychotic behaviors. He proposed three types of anxiety.

1. **Reality anxiety/objective anxiety:** Justifiable fears in the real world like natural disasters, wild animals' and speeding cars, etc.
2. **Neurotic anxiety:** Fear which arouses out of conflict between id and ego, i.e. children are often punished for expressing their sexual and aggressive behaviors; therefore the wish to gratify certain id impulses generates anxiety.
3. **Moral anxiety:** Conflict between the id and superego. Children are punished for violating their parents' moral code and adults are punished for violating society's moral codes.

Freud believed that anxiety serves as warning signal which induces tension and alerts the individual that the ego is being threatened unless action is taken the ego might be overthrown. He postulated several defence mechanisms and noted that we use many defense mechanisms in our day to life to defend ourselves against anxiety.

Freud's Psychosexual Stages of Development

Freud believed that all behaviors are defensive but that not everyone uses the same defenses in the same way. All of us driven by the same id impulses but there is not the same universality in the way ego and superego operates in each individual. Although the structure is same but the content varies from one person to another. Thus our personality is formed on the basis of unique relationships we have as children with various people and objects.

Freud considered childhood experiences shape and crystallize the adult personality. He sensed strong sexual conflicts in the infant and young child, conflicts that seemed to revolve around specific regions of the body. He noted that each body region has greater significance as the center of conflict; each stage is defined by the erogenous zone of the body.

At each stage, a different erogenous zone, or area of the body that produces pleasurable feelings, becomes important and can become the source of conflict. Conflicts that are not fully resolved can result in fixation, or getting stuck in an earlier stage of development. The child may grow into an adult but will still carry emotional and psychological scar from that earlier fixated stage. Because the personality or psyche develops as a result of sexual development, Freud proposed five stages of personality development which is connected to the psychosexual development of the child.

1. **Oral stage (birth to 18 months):** Infants who depend completely on their caregivers to satisfy their needs relieve their sexual tension by sucking and swallowing; when their baby teeth erupt they obtain oral pleasure by chewing and biting. According to Freud, infants who get too much gratification at this stage grow into overly optimistic and dependent adults; those who receive too little may become pessimistic and hostile in later life. Fixation at this stage is linked to several characteristics including lack of confidence, sarcasm and argumentativeness.
2. **Anal stage (18 months to 3 years):** In this stage the major source of pleasure changes from mouth to anal region, the children get pleasure from holding in and excreting feces. In Freud's view if parents are too strict in toilet training, some children may have temper tantrums and may live in self-destructive ways as adults. If parents are too lenient, their children may become messy, unorganized and sloppy.
3. **Phallic stage (3 to 6 years):** When children reach phallic stage after age of 3 years, they discover their genitals and develop marked attachment to the parent of the opposite sex while becoming jealous of the same sex parent. In boys, Freud called this the oedipal complex after the character in Greek, who killed his father and married his mother; whereas for girls, it is Electra complex, involving possessive love for their father and jealousy toward their mother. Fixation at this stage leads to vanity and egotism in adult life.
4. **Latency stage (6 to 12 years):** At the end of the phallic stage children lose interests in sexual behavior and enter into a latency period. During this stage boys play with boys and girls play with girls and neither sex takes much interest in the other.
5. **Genital stage (12 years onwards):** At puberty the individual enters the last stage, sexual impulses and unfulfilled desires from infancy and childhood are satisfied. The focus during this stage is on mature, adult sexuality which Freud defined as sexual intercourse.

Neo-Freudian Psychoanalytic Theory

A series of successors who were trained in traditional Freudian theory but later rejected some of its major points are known as neo-Freudians. Theorists like Carl Jung, Alfred Adler, Karen Horney, Erich Fromm, Henry Murray and Erik Erikson are some of the neo-Freudians. They placed greater emphasis on the functions of ego by insisting that it has more control than the id over day-to-day activities. They focused more on the social environment and minimized the importance of sex as a driving force in people's lives. They stressed upon the effects of society and culture on personality development.

- **Carl Jung's Theory of Personality-Analytical Psychology**
  - Jung created a new and elaborate explanation of human nature which he called analytical psychology. He redefined **libido as a more generalized psychic energy** through which psychological activities such as perceiving, thinking, feeling and wishing are carried out.
  - Jung suggested that we have a **universal collective unconscious**—an inherited set of ideas, feelings, images and symbols that are shared with all humans and our ancestral past. This collective unconscious contains archetypes which have universal symbolic representations of particular types of people, objects or experiences. For example, belief in Supreme Being, love of mother and behavior specific to fear of snakes.
  - Jung divided personality into eight types based on interactions of the attitudes (introversion and extraversion) and the functions (thinking, feeling, sensing and intuiting). (Table 11.4)
- **Alfred Adler's individual psychology:** Alfred Adler was also in disagreement with Freud about the psychosexual development of personality. Adler (1954) developed the theory that as young, helpless children people develop feelings of inferiority complex when comparing themselves to the more powerful, superior adults in their world. The driving force behind all human endeavors, emotions and thoughts was not seeking pleasure but seeking of superiority. The term **inferiority complex** is used to describe adults who have not been able to overcome the feelings of inadequacy they developed as children. He also developed a theory that the **birth order** of the child influences the personality.

- **Karen Horney-psychoanalytic interpersonal theory:** Karen Horney was one of the earliest female psychologists who had disagreements with Freud over the concept of penis envy. She proposed her concept of **womb envy** stating that men felt the need to compensate for their lack of childbearing ability by striving for success in other areas. Horney also focused on personality development in the context of social relationships particularly on **parent and child relationship.** She stressed the importance of **cultural factors in the determination of personality**.
- **Erich Fromm's humanistic psychoanalysis:** A German born American Psychoanalyst developed theories to **integrate psychology with cultural analysis** and Marxist historical materialism. He argued that humanity's separation from the natural world has produced feelings of anxiety, loneliness, isolation and powerlessness. Each socioeconomic class fosters a particular character, governed by ideas that justify it and maintain it. Fromm believed that humans have the ability to shape our personality and society. Life's ultimate, innate goal is the realization of our potentialities and capacities.
- **Henry Murray's theory of personality:** Henry Murray, an American psychologist believed that human behavior may be understood by the **process of satisfying motives and needs**. Personality can be described in terms of these needs and the ways they interact with environmental forces.
- **Erik Erikson's theory of psychosocial development:** Erik Erikson, a German psychoanalyst influenced by Freud's work and developed a psychosocial theory centered on ego. He stressed the role of culture and society and the conflicts that can take place within the ego itself whereas Freud emphasized the conflict between id and superego. According to Erikson's theory, every person must go through series of eight interrelated stages over the entire life cycle. In each stage, person experiences a conflict that serves as a turning point in personality development. Successful dealing with conflict results in psychological strength for the entire life while unsuccessful completion of tasks may have negative consequences on individual's sense of self and identity (Table 11.8 and Fig.11.4).

Table 11.8: Erik Erikson's stages of psychosocial development

Stage and ages	Psychosocial crisis	Virtue/basic strength	Significant relationship	Task	Positive outcome	Negative outcome
Infancy (0–1 year)	Trust vs mistrust	Hope	Mother	Viewing the world as safe and reliable, relationships are nurturing, stable and dependable	Sense of security	Suspiciousness, insecurity, worthlessness
Early childhood (1–3 years)	Autonomy vs shame and doubt	Will	Parents	Achieving a sense of control and free will	Sense of independence	Low self-esteem, feeling shame, dependency on substances and people
Preschool (3–6 years)	Initiative vs guilt	Purpose	Family	Beginning development of a conscience learning to manage conflict and anxiety	Balance between spontaneity and restraint	Passive personality and strong feelings of guilt
School age (6–12 years)	Industry vs inferiority	Competence	Neighbors, school	Emerging confidence in own ability taking pleasure in accomplishments	Sense of self-confidence	Unmotivated and unreliable
Adolescence (12–18 years)	Identity vs role confusion	Fidelity	Peers, role model	Formulating a sense of self and belonging	Sense of self-identity	Rebellion, substance abuse
Early adulthood (18–25 years)	Intimacy vs isolation	Love	Friends, partners	Establishing loving relationships and meaningful attachments to others.	Forming close personal relationship	Emotional immaturity, deny the need for personal relationship
Middle adulthood (25–45 years)	Generativity vs stagnation	Care	Household, workmates	Building family and guiding the next generation	Promoting others well-being	Inability to show concern for anyone but self
Late adulthood/ older adult (45 years-death)	Ego integrity vs despair	Wisdom	Mankind	Accepting responsibility for one's self and life	Sense of satisfaction with life	Has difficulty in dealing with issues of ageing and death, feelings of hopelessness

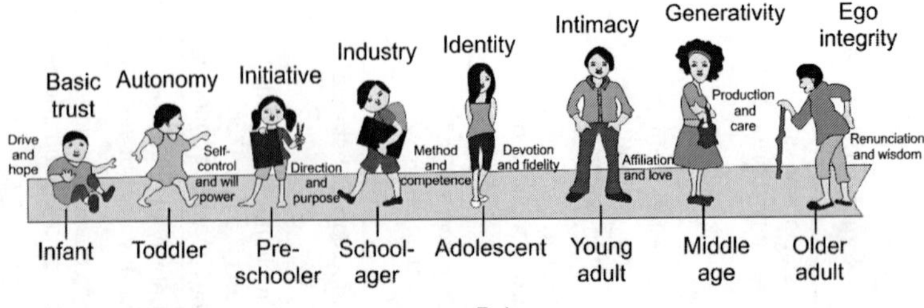

Fig. 11.4: Erikson's stages of psychosocial development

- **Trait and type theories of personality:** Trait is a typical personal characteristics or quality which is displayed in different situations.

  Trait theory is the personality approach that proposes that all people possess certain traits, but the degree to which particular trait applies to a specific person varies and can be counted. For example; people often say—he is kind-hearted, she is really smart, etc. grouping people by traits is made trait approach to personality has been popular for so long.
- **Gordon Allport's theory:** Gordon Allport, an American Psychologist, presented a positive image of human nature and insisted upon the uniqueness of individual. He organized traits into three levels of hierarchy, i. cardinal traits, ii. central traits and iii. secondary traits.
  - **Cardinal traits:** traits which dominate and shape the individuals behavior, e.g. Mother Teresa's selfless service to the mankind. It is at the top of the hierarchy and known as individual's master control. It is considered as an individual's ruling passions. Only few people have personalities dominated by a single trait.
  - **Central trait:** Second level in hierarchy. General characteristics found in a person such as honesty, sociability, kindness, the number may vary from person-to-person. They are the basic building blocks that shape the person's behavior.
  - **Secondary traits:** Bottom level in hierarchy. These are inconsistent and less relevant in reflecting the personality of an individual, not very obvious. For example, a friendly person may get angry when someone tickles him.

- **Raymond Cattell's 16 factor personality theory:** Raymond Cattell, a British psychologist using a statistical method of identifying patterns of behavior which he called factors. According to him, 16 factors or traits are the basic structural units which represent the dimensions of personality. He described that each person contains all 16 traits to a certain degree, but they might be high in some traits and low in others. While all people have some degree of indefinite characteristics. For example; some people might be always worried whereas others are very confident (Table 11.9).

Table 11.9: Cattell's 16 PF trait theory

	Source traits	
Reserved	vs	Outgoing
Less intelligent	vs	More intelligent
Emotionally unstable	vs	Emotionally stable
	Surface traits	
Submissive	vs	Dominant
Serious	vs	Happy-go-lucky
Expedient	vs	Conscientious
Timid	vs	Venturesome
Thought-minded	vs	Sensitive
Trusting	vs	Suspicious
Practical	vs	Imaginative
Forthright	vs	Shrewd
Self assured	vs	Apprehensive
Conservative	vs	Experimenting
Group dependent	vs	Self-sufficient
Undisciplined	vs	Controlled
Relaxed	vs	Tense

- **Hans Eysenck personality theory:** Hans Jurgen Eysenck, German psychologist described one's personality as a hierarchy of traits. He related the personality of an individual to the functioning of the autonomic nervous system. According to Eysenck, personality into three dimensions namely; two dimensions of neuroticism (stable vs unstable), combination of introversion-extroversion (a person's level of sociability), and psychoticism (distorted reality of a person). Eysenck illustrated extroversion and introversion differently, based on the natural states of arousal which means excitation. In keeping with, introverts have higher level of arousal hence they do not need any external stimulating environment whereas extroverts have a lower level of arousal and select environment that give more stimulation.

- **Humanistic approaches of personality:** Humanism, humanistic, humanist are different terminologies used in psychology to describe an approach which studies the human being as a whole person and the uniqueness of each individual. Humanistic approach is also called phenomenological meaning personality is studied from the view of individual's subjective experience. Humanists focus on the here and now rather than past or future. The theory stresses the person worth of an individual, the centrality of human values and the creative, nature of human beings. Humanistic theorists like Carl Rogers and Abraham Maslow denied the internal conflicts of Freud's view and the mechanistic view of behaviorism.
  - **Carl Rogers person centered approach:** Carl Rogers, an influential American psychologist, one of the founding fathers of psychotherapy developed a theory that stressed the importance of self-actualizing tendency in shaping human personality. He believed that human beings are constantly reacting to stimuli with their subjective reality field which he called phenomenological field which changes constantly. In due course, an individual develops a self-concept based on the feedback from this field of reality. Rogers defined self-concept as 'the organized, consistent set of perceptions and beliefs about oneself'. This consists of all the ideas and values that explain what I am and what I can do. Rogers also insisted upon unconditional positive regard or unconditional love. Positive regard is a need for acceptance, love and approval from others especially from the mother during infancy. In unconditional positive regard, the mother's love and approval are given freely and are not conditional on the child's behavior. Once we internalize the attitudes of others, positive regard comes from ourselves.

He listed seven characteristics of fully functioning person who represents the peak of psychological development.

1. A growing openness to experience
2. An increasing existential lifestyle—living each moment fully
3. Increasing orgasmic trust
4. Freedom of choice
5. Higher levels of creativity
6. Reliability and constructiveness
7. A rich full life.

– **Abraham Maslow's hierarchy of needs:** Abraham Maslow an American psychologist created his theory based on the hierarchy of human needs. He argued that each person is born with instinctual needs that lead to growth, development and actualization. The hierarchy of needs include physiological needs (for food, water, air, sleep and sex) and the needs for safety, belongingness and love, self-esteem and self-actualization. Maslow stated that people are motivated to achieve certain needs and some needs take lead over others. When one need is fulfilled a person seeks to fulfil the next one and so on. Every person is capable and has the desire to move up the hierarchy toward a level of self-actualization. Maslow viewed human nature is optimistic, emphasizing-free will, conscious choice, uniqueness, the ability to overcome childhood experiences and innate goodness. Personality is influenced both by heredity and by environment and the ultimate goal is self-actualization.

- **Behavioral and social learning approaches of personality:** Behavioral theorists describe personality is simply an aggregation of learned responses to stimuli, sets of overt behaviors or habit systems. Personality refers only to what can be objectively observed and manipulated.

  – **BF Skinner approach to personality:** Burrhus Frederic Skinner, an American psychologist tried to understand personality through laboratory research. He denied the existence of an entity called personality and personality is simply a pattern of operant behaviors. He believed that differences' in learning experiences are the main reason for individual differences in behavior. These patterns of behavior are learnt either directly (reward as positive reinforcement of good behavior or punishment as a negative reinforcement of bad behavior) or indirectly (through observational learning or modelling). Skinner insisted that our behavior and personality traits can be shaped and controlled by the environment, hence if the negative traits to be changed into positive, the environment to be modified.

- **N Miller and J Dollard approach to personality:** John Dollard and Neal Miller, American psychologists used principles of learning to explain complex human behavior. In their view, habits makeup the structure of personality. They believe that habits (a deeply grained, learned pattern of response) are governed by four elements of learning.
  1. Drive any intense stimulus strong enough to lead a person to action or motivates the response, e.g. hunger, pain, lust, etc.
  2. Cue-external stimuli or signs that guide responses or elicit the response, e.g. red traffic light is a cue to stop whereas green is a cue to go.
  3. Responses—any behavior observable or internal.
  4. Reward—reinforcement.
- **Albert Bandura's social learning theory:** Albert Bandura, an American psychologist believed that human behaviors and personality is developed through the social experiences. He focused on the acquisition and modification of personality traits through observational learning or modelling or imitation which has a significant role in determining subsequent behavior.

• **Biological and evolutionary approaches to personality:** Biological and evolutionary approaches suggest that important components of personality are inherited. The field of behavioral genetics is devoted to the study of how much of an individual's personality is due to inherited traits. These approaches' argue that personality is determined at least in part by our genes in the same way our height is determined.

PSYCHOMETRIC ASSESSMENT OF PERSONALITY

Assessment simply means to measure, to test or to evaluate. Psychological assessment is an objective and standardized measure of an individual's behavioral characteristics'.

Psychometric is the field of study related to the theory and technique of psychological measurement which measures knowledge, attitudes, personality traits, etc.

Personality test is a questionnaire or other standardized instrument designed to reveal aspects of an individual's character or psychological makeup.

Importance of Personality Assessment

In 1920, the first personality tests were developed in order to ease the personnel selection in army. Personality assessment is carried out for different reasons.

- To describe human character in quantifiable forms.
- To refine clinical diagnosis
- To structure and inform psychological interventions
- To increase the accuracy of behavioral predictions in a variety of contexts and settings. For example, clinical, forensic, organizational, and educational.

Types of Personality Assessment Tests

Methods of assessing personality vary according to the theory of personality, however most professionals take more of a eclectic view of personality. Some of the commonly used methods are (Table 11.10).

Table 11.10: Types of personality assessment

Type of assessment	Mostly used by
Interviews	Psychoanalysts, human therapists
Behavioral assessments • Direct observation • Rating scales • Frequency counts	Behaviorqal and sociocognitive therapists
Projective tests • Rorschach inkblot test • Thematic apperception test • Children apperception test • Word association test • Sentence completion test	Psychoanalysts
Personality inventories • Minnesota multiphase personality Inventory (MMPI) • 16 personality factor questionnaire (16 PF)	Trait theorists

Interview Method

It is a method of personality assessment in which a professional asks questions to the client and allows the client to answer. It gives opportunities for mutual exchange of ideas and informations between the subject and therapist. Structured interview adopts a systematic and predefined approach to a specific situation (Table 11.11). Usually, a professional have a list of fixed or predetermined set of questions and play a passive role in the interview. A predefined set of guidelines or question will help the professional to lead on to complete the requirement and stick to the topic throughout interview.

Table 11.11: Structured interview vs unstructured interview

Structured interview	Unstructured Interview
• Is a formal interview are like a job interview • Adopts a systematic and predetermined approach to the specific situation	• An informal interview is like a casual conversation or open interrogation • There are no set of questions
• Here the interview is definite or specific what traits or personality need to assessed	• The interviewer can ask any question on the subject relevant to the situation. (free to drift to explore specific information)
• Usually a list of fixed, predetermined set of questions, are prepared based on the criteria or specific set to be requirement	• Interview should not restrict to a set of particular set of predetermined questions
• The interviewer stays within their role and maintains social distance from the interviewee	• Participant is given the opportunity to raise whatever topics he/she feels are relevant and ask them in their own way
• Every participant is encountered in the same order and in the same way in the assessment of the specific set of traits or behavior	• Here in this type qualitative or descriptive data is likely to be collected

Behavioral Assessments

Behavioral theorists do not want to typically look into the mind. They assume that personality is learned responses to stimuli in the environment.

- **Direct observation method:** This is to observe a person's actions in day-to-day situations over a long period preferably in a natural setting of home, school, and workplace. Observation allows them to see how situation and environment interact to influence the behavior. It is an expensive and time-consuming method, may also yield faulty results whenever the presence of the observer affects people's behavior.

- **Situational test:** In this type situations are artificially created in which an individual is asked to do some acts which are related to the personality traits under testing. For example, to test the work ability of a staff nurse, some situations can be created to check the competency.
- **Rating scale:** Here, numerical rating is assigned either by the assessor or by client for specific behaviors.
- **Frequency counts:** The assessor literally counts the frequency of certain behaviors' within a specific time limit. Educators make use of both rating scales and frequency counts to diagnose behavioral problems such as attention deficit, social skill at various levels, etc.

Projective Tests

It is a personality test in which words, images, situations are presented to a person and asked to give unlimited responses or interpretations in order to analyze the unconscious expression of elements of personality. It is based on Freud's psychoanalytical theory.

Assumptions of projective tests

- The more unstructured the stimuli the more the clients reveal about their personality
- Every response gives meaning for analysis of personality
- There is an unconscious attempt of giving the answers
- Clients unaware of what they disclose during test.

Types of Projective Tests

Rorschach Inkblot Test

It is the one of the most frequently used projective personality tests named after Hermann Rorschach; a Swiss psychiatrist interpreted the inkblots as a key to personality. This test involves 10 cards with unique inkblot design in each card. Client is asked specific what they see in each blot. The test instructions are minimal so the responses will be completely their own. After, interpreting all the blots the person goes over the cards again with the therapist and explains which part of each blot prompted each response. Therapists score responses on key factors such as reference to color, shape, figures seen in blot and responses to the whole or to detail (Fig. 11.5).

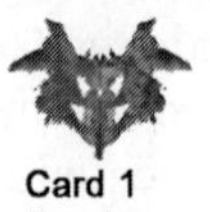

Card 1
Popular responses bat, butterfly, moth

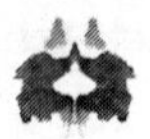

Card 2
Popular responses two humans, four-legged animal, dog, elephant, bear

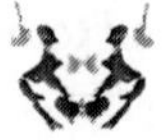

Card 3
Popular responses two humans, human figures

Card 4
Popular responses animal hide, skin, rug

Card 5
Popular responses bat, butterfly, moth

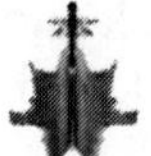

Card 6
Popular responses animal hide, skin, rug

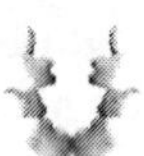

Card 7
Popular responses human heads or faces

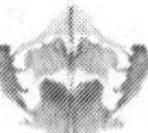

Card 8
Popular responses animal: not cat or dog four-legged animal

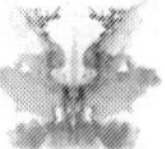

Card 9
Popular responses human

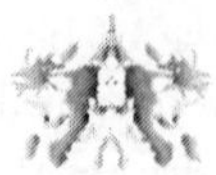

Card 10
Popular responses crab, lobster, spider rabbit head, caterpillars, worms, snakes

Fig. 11.5: Rorschach inkblot test

Thematic Apperception Test (TAT)

It was developed by Henry Murray and his colleagues using 20 pictures of all black and white cards with people in ambiguous situations as the visual stimuli. The client is asked to create a complete story about the person or people in the picture, including what led up the scene depicted, what characters are doing at the moment, what their thoughts and feelings are and what the outcome will be. The story is interpreted by the psychoanalyst, who looks for revealing statements and projection of client's own problem onto the people in the pictures (Fig. 11.6).

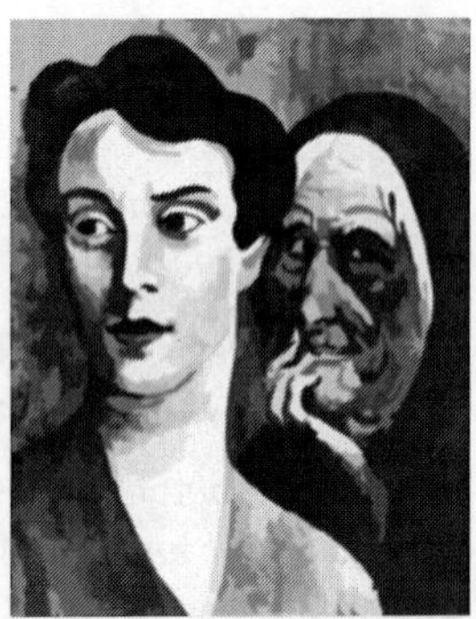

Fig. 11.6: Thematic apperception test

Children Apperception Test (CAT)

This projective test is developed for children of both sexes, between 3 to 10 years of age by Dr Leopald Bellak. This test consists of 10 cards with pictures of animals instead of human characters. These animals are in various real life situations. The child is asked to describe the situations and makeup stories about the animals in the picture, and the psychoanalysts interpret the psychosexual conflicts related to certain stages of child's development.

Word Association Test

It was developed as a research instrument by Francis Galton and was subsequently Carl Jung developed as a clinical diagnostic tool. In this test therapist will say to the client a hundred series of stimulus words one word at a time. The client should immediately say the first word which comes to his or her mind. There is no right or wrong answers. The therapist records the reply to each word given by the client. The reaction time and unusual speech or behavior accompanying the responses will also be noted. Based on the client's responses the personality will be determined.

Sentence Completion Test

It is a semistructured projective test, consists of list of open-ended, incomplete sentences, called stems. The client is asked to go through the list and complete the sentences in ways that are meaningful to them. For example, I am worried over........., I feel proud when..........., my hero is.........interpretation of response is highly subjective however, it is superior than word association test because the client can give more than one word to complete the sentence.

Personality Inventories

Trait theorists are typically more interested in using personality inventories. It is a questionnaire that has a standard list of questions and only requires certain specific answers such as yes or no or cannot decide. There are number of questionnaires used in psychology for counseling and research work. They are also used in staff selection for employment and promotion.

- **Minnesota multiphas personality inventory (MMPI):** Originally developed by Starke R Hathaway and JC McKinley to test adult personality and psychopathology. It is one of most widely used and researched standardized tools. The MMPI has about

567 true or false questions to rule out abnormal human behavior. Some of the statements include:
  - I like machine
  - I get angry sometimes
  - I am an important person
- **16 personality factor questionnaire (16 PF):** Raymond B Cattell developed 16 PF inventory using 16 personality traits. It consists of 164 statements about on a scale of 1 (disagree), 2 (slightly disagree), 3 (neither agree nor disagree), 4 (slightly agree) and 5 (agree).

ALTERATIONS IN PERSONALITY

In most theories, the static content and structural aspects of personality are primary and therefore personality change is difficult problem. Personality can be altered due to mainly two reasons; physical and mental illness.

Behavioral Changes due to Illness

Behavior may vary from person to person when an individual encounter illness. It is affected by many variables like age, sex, occupation, socioeconomic status, etc. Behavioral changes due to short-term illness are mild and short lived. On the other end, certain personality types itself can predisposes an individual to certain illness or prolong the illness state. Some of the abnormal behavior can be manifested during physical illness include:
- Uncooperativeness
- Disorganized speech and behavior
- Confusion and delirium
- Withdrawn behavior
- Hostility
- Shame and guilt
- Mood swings.

An individual may have more than one type of change. For example, person with confusion due to Alzheimer's disease sometimes become depressed, and person with delirium may have disorganized speech.

Behavioral Changes due to Personality Disorders

Personality disorders diagnosed when the abnormal behaviors overtly evident and cause significant social and occupational dysfunction and subjective distress.

Personality disorders differ from personality change in their timing and the mode of occurrence. These are developmental conditions, which occurs in childhood or adolescence and continue in adulthood. They are not secondary to another mental disorder or brain disease but they may coexist with other illness.

Table 11.12: Overview of personality disorders

Category	Personality disorder	Signs and symptoms
Cluster A (suspicious)	Paranoid personality disorder	• Extremely distrustful and suspicious • Thinks other people are lying to them or trying to manipulate them • Thinks there are hidden meanings in remarks • Tendency to hold grudges • Worries that their partner is unfaithful
	Schizoid personality disorder	• Detachment and social withdrawal • Disinterested in forming close relationships with other people including family • Prefers to be alone with their own thoughts • Limited range of emotional expression • Inability to take pleasure in most of the activities
	Dissocial personality disorder/ antisocial personality disorder	• Chronic antisocial activities that violate the rights of others • Consistently irresponsible • Aggressive behavior • Recurring problems with the law • Consistently irresponsible • Lack of remorse for behavior
Cluster B (emotional impulsive)	Histrionic personality disorder	• Constantly seeking attention • Excessively emotional, dramatic or sexually provocative to gain attention • Easily influenced by others • Excessive concern with physical appearance
	Narcissistic personality disorder	• Self-centered, self-absorbed • Lacking in empathy for others • Fantasy about power, success and attractive-ness • Exaggeration of achievements and talents • Arrogance
	Emotionally unstable personality disorder	**Impulsive type** • Emotional instability • Lack of impulse control • Outbursts of violence and threatening behaviors in response to criticism by others

Contd...

Contd...

Category	Personality disorder	Signs and symptoms
		Borderline type • Disturbed self-image • Chronic feelings of emptiness • Involvement in intense and unstable relationship leading to repeated emotional crises • Excessive effort to avoid abandonment • Repeated suicidal threats and act
Cluster C (anxious)	Anxious personality disorder	• Appears painfully shy, socially inhibited • Feels inadequate and extremely sensitive to rejection • Lacks confidence to establish relationship
	Dependent personality disorder	• Inability to be independent • Excessive need for others to look after them • Unable to make decisions without others guidance • Inability to express disagreement with others • Lack of confidence
	Anankastic personality disorder	• Preoccupied with orderliness and ways to control their environment • Excessive interest in lists, timetables and rules • Pervasive desire for perfection • Being unable to delegate tasks to others

The exact cause for personality disorder is unknown. But it is hypothesized that genetic, biological, social, developmental, psychological and environmental factors have significant role in determining the personality disorders. Personality change is acquired usually during adult life following severe or prolonged stress, extreme environmental deprivation, chronic mental illness, brain disease or injury. Table 11.12 give a brief overview about different personality disorders.

PERSONALITY AND NURSING

- **Understanding and treating psychopathology:** Psychoanalysis, psychodynamic therapy, behavioral therapy, and humanistic counseling are all different approaches used to treat patients with various psychopathological dysfunctions.
- **Personality testing in everyday life:** Most people enjoy finding out something about themselves. People want to know what I am really like. What is my personality? There are number of online personality tests available on the internet. Although all

tests are not equal in quality, reliability or validity. As these tests lack professional interpretation and one must use it properly.

- **Understanding personality types in workplace:** Knowing one's own personality allows them to work in an environment more effectively. Thus helping the person to avoid conflicts, appreciate diversity, improving decision making skills in the workplace.
- **Recruitment process:** Personality inventories are widely used in selection of employees in organization.
- **Education and training:**
  - Provide students with new awareness of their strengths and the differences they might have with their friends, teachers and parents.
  - An understanding of personality helps the nurse to predict the behavior of self and others.
  - It is essential that nurse should develop a pleasing and strong personality to be successful in profession.
  - When working healthcare team, it is important that the nurse should possess interpersonal skills in order to deliver quality patient care services.
  - The personality construct lifestyle of the nurse plays an important role in stress management and burnout.
  - Nurses should be very careful not to use stereotypical explanations when working with individuals who have physical, mental and other life changing experiences. If the nurse understands that the way an individual behaves is a consequence of their personality, definitely the nurse accepts that they are unlikely to change.

Suggested Reading

- Ciccarelli SK, Meyer GE. Psychology South Edition. Pearson Education, 2015; p 476.
- Feldman RS. Essentials of Understanding Psychology. 11th ed, McGraw Hill Education; p 380.
- Morris CG, Maisto AA, Misra G. Psychology for Nurses. Pearson Education, 2010; pp 160-61.
- Schultz DP, Schultz SE.Theories of Personality, 8th ed. Thomson Educational Publishing.
- Sreevani R. Psychology for Nurses. 2nd ed. Jaypee Brothers Medical Publishers (P) Ltd., New Delhi, 2013; p 126.

REVIEW QUESTIONS

SHORT-ESSAY TYPE QUESTIONS

1. Define personality. Discuss the factors affecting personality.
2. Discuss various method of personality assessment.
3. Discuss the psychoanalysis approach of personality in detail.

MULTIPLE CHOICE QUESTIONS

1. Which of the following personality traits very much related to sanguine personality?
   a. Reserved
   b. Calm
   c. Sociable
   d. Pessimistic
2. Which of the following personality structure related with pleasure seeking?
   a. Id
   b. Ego
   c. Superego
   d. Unconscious mind
3. TAT a method of personality assessment belong to which of the following category?
   a. Survey method
   b. Projective technique
   c. Personality inventory
   d. Questionnaire method
4. Which of the following personality assessment method was proposed by Cattell?
   a. Rorschach Inkblot method
   b. Sentence completion inventory
   c. 16 Personality factors
   d. Color drawing method
5. Thematic Apperception test was developed by:
   a. Hermann Rorschach
   b. Henry A Murray
   c. Funder
   d. Sigmund Freud
6. It consist storage of major portion of memory, sensation, thought and experiences.
   a. Conscious brain
   b. Unconscious brain
   c. Subconscious brain
   d. Both a & b
7. Ego begins to develop at the age of:
   a. Birth
   b. 1–2 months of life
   c. 4–6 months of life
   d. 3–4 years of life

8. Psychoanalysis approach was proposed by following:
   a. Carl Jung
   b. BF Skinner
   c. Sigmund Freud
   d. Ivan Pavlov
9. Oedipus complex develops during which of the following psychosexual stage of development given by S Freud?
   a. Oral
   b. Anal
   c. Phallic
   d. Latency
10. According to Erik Erikson's stages of Psychosocial Development, Gender identity vs Role confusion phenomena occur in which of the following developmental stage?
    a. Infancy
    b. Early childhood
    c. School age
    d. Adolescence
11. Personality traits theory was proposed by:
    a. Carl Jung
    b. Gordon Allport
    c. Sigmund Freud
    d. Ivan Pavlov
12. 16 PF study is the part of:
    a. Behavioral technique
    b. Projective technique
    c. Related personality test
    d. Personality inventory

ANSWER KEY

1.	c	2.	a	3.	b	4.	c	5.	b	6.	b	7.	c
8.	c	9.	c	10.	d	11.	b	12.	d				

Developmental Psychology

Chapter 12

INTRODUCTION

Human life starts from a single fertilized cell. This cell is under constant interaction with the environment. There are various changes take place in this cell in mother's womb and after birth in the world. This changes leads to the growth and development of the child.

Growth and development usually referred to as a unit, express the sum of the numerous changes that take place during the lifetime of an individual. The entire course is a dynamic process that encompasses several interrelated dimensions.

- **Growth:** An increase in number and size of cells as they divide and synthesize new proteins; results in increased size and weight of the whole or any of its parts.
- **Development:** A gradual change and expansion; advancement from lower to more advanced stages of complexity; the emerging and expanding of the individual's capacities through growth, maturation, and learning.
- **Maturation:** Refers to an increase in functionality of various body systems or developmental skills.

All of these processes are interrelated, simultaneous, and ongoing; none occurs apart from the others. The processes depend on a sequence of endocrine, genetic, constitutional, environmental, and nutritional influences. The child's body becomes larger and more complex; the personality simultaneously expands in scope and complexity. Very simply, growth can be viewed as a quantitative change and development as a qualitative change (Table 12.1).

PATTERNS OF GROWTH AND DEVELOPMENT

There are definite and predictable patterns in growth and development that are continuous, orderly, and progressive. These patterns or trends are universal and basic to all human beings, but each human being accomplishes these in a manner and time unique to that individual.

Table 12.1: Growth and development comparison

Growth	Development
• Growth refers to increase in physical aspects of the organism	• Development refers to overall changes in the whole of the organism
• Growth is structural	• Development is functional
• Growth is quantitative	• Development is qualitative
• Growth is cellular	• Development is organizational
• Growth stops when the organism reaches the stage of maturity	• Development is a lifelong process
• Growth involves body changes	• Development involves changes from origin to maturity
• Growth influences the process of development, but not always	• Development occurs without growth

- **Directional patterns:** Growth and development precede in regular, related directions or gradients and reflect the physical development and maturation of neuromuscular functions. The first pattern is the *cephalocaudal*, or head-to-tail direction. Whereas the head end of the organism develops first and is large and complex, the lower end is small and simple and takes shape at a later period.

Second, the *proximodistal*, or near-to-far, trend applies to the midline-to-peripheral concept. These trends or patterns are bilateral and appear symmetric—each side develops in the same direction and at the same rate as the other.

The third pattern, *differentiation*, describes development from simple operations to more complex activities and functions. From broad, global patterns of behavior, more specific, refined patterns emerge. All areas of development (physical, mental, social, and emotional) proceed in this direction.

Table 12.2: Theories of psychological development

Theory	Theorist
• Psychosexual development	• Sigmund Freud
• Psychosocial development	• Erik Erikson
• Interpersonal theory	• Sullivan
• Theory of object relations	• Mahler
• Cognitive development	• Jean Piaget
• Moral judgment	• Kohlberg
• Spiritual development	• Fowler

- **Sequential patterns:** In all dimensions of growth and development, there is a definite, predictable sequence, with each child normally passing through every stage. Children crawl before they creep, creep before they stand, and stand before they walk.

Later facets of the personality are built on the early foundation of trust. The child babbles, then forms words, and finally sentences; writing emerges from scribbling.

STAGE OF GROWTH AND DEVELOPMENT AND TASKS

Developmental stages are identified by age. Behaviors can then be evaluated for age-appropriateness. Ideally, an individual successfully fulfills all the tasks associated with one stage before moving on to the next stage (at the appropriate age). Realistically, however, this seldom happens. Stages overlap, and an individual may be working on tasks associated with several stages at one time. Some of the developmental tasks in different age group are as follows:

Table 12.3: Freud's stages of psychosexual development

Age	Stage	Major developmental tasks
Birth to 18 months	Oral	Relief from anxiety through oral gratification of needs
18 months to 3 years	Anal	Learning independence and control, with focus on the excretory function
3–6 years	Phallic	Identification with parent of the same sex; development of sexual identity; focus on genital organs
6–12 years	Latency	Sexuality repressed; focus on relationships with same sex peers
13–20 years	Genital	Libido reawakened as genital organs mature; focus on relationships with members of the opposite sex

Table 12.4: Stages of development in Sullivan's interpersonal theory

Age	Stage	Major developmental tasks
Birth to 18 months	Infancy	Relief from anxiety through oral gratification of needs
18 months to 6 years	Childhood	Learning to experience a delay in personal gratification without undue anxiety
6–9 years	Juvenile	Learning to form satisfactory peer relationships
9–12 years	Preadolescence	Learning to form satisfactory relationships with persons of same gender initiating feelings of affection for another person
12–14 years	Early adolescence	Learning to form satisfactory relationships with persons of the opposite gender; developing a sense of identity
14–21 years	Late adolescence	Establishing self-identity; experiencing satisfying relationships; working to develop a lasting, intimate opposite-gender relationship

Table 12.5: Stages of development in Erikson's psychosocial theory

Age	Stage	Major developmental tasks
0–18 months (infant)	Trust vs mistrust	To develop a basic trust in the mothering figure and be able to generalize it to others
18 months to 3 years (toddler)	Autonomy vs shame and doubt	To gain some self-control and independence within the environment
3–6 years (preschooler)	Initiative vs guilt	To develop a sense of purpose and the ability to initiate and direct own activities
6–12 years (school age)	Industry vs inferiority	To achieve a sense of self-confidence by learning, competing, performing successfully, and receiving recognition from significant others, peers, and acquaintances
12–20 years (adolescents)	Identity vs role confusion	To integrate the tasks mastered in the previous stages into a secure sense of self
20–30 years (early adulthood)	Intimacy vs isolation	To form an intense, lasting relationship or a commitment to another person, cause, institution, or creative effort
30–65 years (late adulthood)	Generativity vs stagnation	To achieve the life goals established for oneself, while also considering the welfare of future generations
65 years to death (old age)	Ego integrity vs despair	To review one's life and derive meaning from both positive and negative events, while achieving a positive sense of self-worth

Table 12.6: Stages of development in Mahler's theory of object relation

Age	Stage	Major developmental tasks
Birth to 1 month	Normal autism	Fulfillment of basic needs for survival and comfort
1–5 months	Symbiosis	Development of awareness of external source of need fulfillment
5–10 months	Separation-individuation (Phase–Differentiation)	Commencement of a primary recognition of separateness from the mothering figure
10–16 months	Separation-individuation (Phase—Practicing)	Increased independence through locomotor functioning; increased sense of separateness of self
16–24 months	Separation-individuation (Phase—Rapprochement)	Acute awareness of separateness of self; learning to seek 'emotional refueling' from mothering figure to maintain feeling of security
24–36 months	Separation-individuation (Phase—Consolidation)	Sense of separateness established; on the way to object constancy (i.e. able to internalize a sustained image of loved object/person when it is out of sight); resolution of separation anxiety

Table 12.7: Stages of development in Piaget's cognitive development

Age	Stage	Major developmental tasks
0–2 years	Sensorimotor	During the first stage, children learn entirely through the movements they make and the sensations that result. They learn: • That they exist separately from the objects and people around them • That they can cause things to happen • That things continue to exist even when they cannot see them
2–7 years	Preoperational	Once children acquire language, they are able to use symbols (such as words or pictures) to represent objects. Their thinking is still very egocentric though–they assume that everyone else sees things from the same viewpoint as they do. They are able to understand concepts like counting, classifying according to similarity, and past-present-future but generally they are still focused primarily on the present and on the concrete, rather than the abstract
7–11 years	Concrete operational	At this stage, children are able to see things from different points of view and to imagine events that occur outside their own lives. Some organized, logical thought processes are now evident and they are able to: • Order objects by size, color gradient, etc. • Understand that if 3 + 4 = 7 then 7 – 4 = 3 • Understand that a red square can belong to both the 'red' category and the 'square' category • Understand that a short wide cup can hold the same amount of liquid as a tall thin cup However, thinking still tends to be tied to concrete reality
11–15 years	Formal operation	Around the onset of puberty, children are able to reason in much more abstract ways and to test hypotheses using systematic logic. There is a much greater focus on possibilities and on ideological issues.

PRINCIPLES OF GROWTH AND DEVELOPMENT

The process of development has been studied experimentally and otherwise. The studies and researches have highlighted certain significant facts or principles underlying this process. Some of the principles of growth and development are elucidated here:

- **Developmental pattern:** Peculiar of the species development occurs in orderly manner and follows a certain sequence. For example, the human body cuts his molars before his incisors,

Table 12.8: Stages of development in Kohlberg's moral development

Level	Age	Stage	Major developmental tasks
Pre-conventional morality	Infancy	Punishment/ obedience	No difference doing right thing and avoiding punishment
	Preschool	Self-interest	Interest shift to rewards rather than punishment-effort is made to secure greatest benefit for oneself
Conventional morality	School age	Conformity and interpersonal accord	The 'good boy/girl' level. Effort is made to secure approval and maintain friendly relations with others
	School age	Authority and social order (law and order)	Orientation toward fixed rules. The purpose of morality is maintaining the social order. Interpersonal accord is expanded to include entire society
Post-conventional morality	Adolescence	Social contract	Mutual benefit, reciprocity. Morally right and legally right are always not same. Utilitarian rules that make life better for everyone
	Adulthood	Universal principles	Morality is based on the principles that transcend mutual benefit

Table 12.9: Stages of development in Fowler's spiritual development

Age	Stage	Major developmental tasks
Infant	Undifferentiated	Trust, hope and love compete with environmental inconsistencies or threat of abandonment
Toddler-preschooler	Intuitive-projective	Initiates parental behavior and attitude about religion and spirituality. Has no real understanding about spiritual concepts
School age	Mythical-literal faith	• Accepts existence of deity • Religious or moral belief are symbolized by stories • Appreciates others' viewpoint • Accepts concept of reciprocal fairness
Adolescents	Synthetic-convention	Questions values and religious belief in an attempt to form own identity
Young adult	Individuating-reflexive	Assume responsibility for own attitude and belief
Late adulthood	Conjunctive faith	Integrates others perspective about faith into own definition of truth
Old age	Universalizing faith	Make concept of love and justice tangible

can stand before he walks and can draw, a circle before he can draw a square. In physical development one can see the cephalocaudal sequence in the prenatal life of the human child. This mean that control of the body as well as improvements in the structure itself develops first in the head and progresses later to parts further from the bread.

The cephalocaudal sequence may be illustrated by the development of motor functions. When the baby is placed in a prone position, he can lift his head by his neck before he can do to by lifting his chest. The control of muscles of the trunk precedes that of the muscles of the arms and legs. Even the specific phases of development such as motor, social and play follows a pattern also. Group play activity follows the self-centered play activity. The child is interested in himself first before he can develop interest in other children. He babbles before he talks, he is dependent on others before he achieves dependence on self.

- **Development proceeds from general to specific responses:** It moves from a generalized to localized behavior. This can be observed in the behavior of infants and young children. Newborn infant moves his whole body at one time instead of moving only one part of it. In the emotional field, the baby first responds to all strange objects with a general fear. Gradually, his fear becomes specific. He reaches out for the object as a whole before he can hold its specific parts.
- **Development is a continuous process:** Development does not occur in parts. Although, it is suggested that there are definite developmental stages such as 'gang age' or 'adolescence', yet it is a fact that growth continues from the moments of conception until the individual's reaches maturity. It takes place at a slow regular pace rather than by 'leaps and bounds'. Development of both physical and mental traits continues gradually until these traits reach their maximum growth.

  For example, speech does not come over-night. It develops gradually from the cries and other sounds made by the baby at birth. The first teeth seem to appear suddenly, but they start developing as early as the fifth fetal month: they cut through the gums about five months after birth. There may be a break in the continuity of growth due to illness, starvation or malnutrition or other environmental factors or some abnormal conditions in the child life.

- **Tempo of growth is not even:** There are periods of accelerated growth and periods of accelerated growth. During infancy and the early preschool years, growth moves swiftly. Later on it slackens growth from 3–6 years is rapid but not as rapid as from birth to 3 years. In early adolescence it is again rapid as compared to the period covering 8–12 years.
- **Different aspects of growth develop at different rates:** Neither all parts of the body grow at the same rate, nor do all aspects of mental growth proceed equally. They reach maturity at different times. For example, the brain attains its mature size around the age of six to eight years. Reasoning and intelligence reaches its peak at a defined age.
- **Most traits are correlated in development:** Generally it is seen that the child whose intellectual development is above average is so in health size, sociability and special aptitudes. Mental defectives tend to be smaller in stature than the normal child. Idiots and imbeciles are often the smallest of the feeble-minded group. There is a correlation between high intelligence and sexual maturity.
- **Growth is complex:** 'It is impossible to understand the physical child without understanding him at the same time as a child who thinks and has feeling'. His mental development is intimately related to his physical growth and its needs. Again, a physical defect may be responsible for the development certain attitudes and social adjustments.
- **Growth is the product of the interaction of heredity and environment:** Neither heredity alone, nor the mere environment is the potent factor in the development of an individual. Hereditary and environment play an important role in growth of an individual. These two work hand in hand from the very conceptions.
- **Each individual grows in his unique ways:** It is definitely indicated in various studies that the differences in physical and mental structure is vary from one individual to another. These individual differences are result of differences in hereditary endowment and environmental exposure. Genetic codes and environmental exposure make every individual to grow in different manner.
- **Growth is both qualitative and quantitative:** Improvement in size and complexity in functions are two inseparable aspects.

Change in size and shape and development complexity in functions occurs simultaneously. *Breckenridge* and *Vincent* have given a nice example to illustrate this principle. The baby's digestive tract not only grows in size, but also changes in structure, permitting digestion of more complex foods and increasing its efficiency in converting foods into simpler forms which the body can use. The younger the child, simpler the emotions in child. With growth, there is an increase of experiences and these produce more and more complex emotional reactions to more and more complicated situations.

- **Development is predictable:** We have seen that the rate of development for each child is fairly constant. The consequence is that it is possible for us to predict at an early age the range within which the mature development of the child is likely to fall. But it may be noted that all types of development, particularly mental development, cannot be predicted with the same degree of accuracy. It is more easily predictable for children whose mental development falls within the normal range rather than for those whose mental development shows marked deviation from the average.

FACTORS AFFECTING GROWTH AND DEVELOPMENT

The integrated nature of growth and development is largely maintained by a constant interaction of genes, hormones, nutrients and other factors. There are several factors which directly or indirectly influence the growth and development of an organism. There are as follows:

- **Heredity:** Heredity is a biological process through which the transmission of physical and social characteristics takes place from parents to offsprings. It greatly influences the different aspects of growth and development, i.e. height, weight and structure of the body, color of hair and eye, intelligence, aptitudes and instincts. However environment equally influences the above aspects in many cases. Biologically speaking heredity is the sum total of traits potentially present in the fertilized ovum (combination of sperm cell and egg cell), by which offsprings are resemblance to their parents and foreparents.
- **Environment:** Environment plays an important role in human life. Psychologically a person's environment consists of the sum total of the stimulations (physical and psychological) which

he receives from his conception. There are different types of environment such as physical, environment, social environment and psychological environment.

- **Physical environment** consists of all outer physical surroundings both in-animate and animate which have to be manipulated in order to provide food, clothing and shelter. Geographical conditions, i.e. weather and climates are physical environment which has considerable impact on individual child.
- **Social environment** is constituted by the society-individuals and institutions, social laws, customs by which human behavior is regulated.
- **Psychological environment** is rooted in individual's reaction with an object. One's love, affection and fellow feeling attitude will strengthen human bond with one another.

So growth and development are regulated by the environment of an individual where he lives.

- **Gender:** Gender acts as an important factor of growth and development. There is difference in growth and development of boys and girls. The boys are generally taller, courageous than the girls but girls show rapid physical growth in adolescence and excel boys. In general the body constitution and structural growth of girls are different from boys. The functions of boys and girls are also different in nature.
- **Nutrition:** Growth and development of the child mainly depend on his food habits and nutrition. The malnutrition has adverse effect on the structural and functional development of the child.
- **Race:** The racial factor has a great influence on height, weight, color, features and body constitution. A child of white race will be white and tall even hair and eye color, facial structure are governed by the same race.
- **Exercise:** Repeated play and exercise play important role in growth and development. It is a fact that repeated play and rest build the strength of the muscle. The increase in muscular strength is mainly due to better circulation and oxygen supply.
- **Hormones:** There are a number of endocrine glands inside the human body. These glands produce one or more hormones. A balance of hormones controls development in the direction of masculinity and that of female hormones steers it toward

feminist. These hormones play important role in growth and development at different stage of human being. Under secretion and over secretions of hormones affect the growth and development accordingly.

- **Learning and reinforcement:** Learning is the most important and fundamental topic in the whole science of psychology. Development consists of maturation and learning. Without any learning the human organism is a structure of various limbs, all other internal organs with muscles and bones. Reinforcement helps in learning. Reinforcement could be physical, psychological, and financial.

PSYCHOLOGICAL NEEDS OF DIFFERENT AGE GROUP PEOPLE

Developmental psychology is concerned with the scientific understanding of age-related changes in experience and behavior. At each stage, individual need different desire and their fulfillment. Unfulfillment of these needs leads frustration in a particular individual. It is important to identify these developmental needs in order to give meaning to life.

Following are the psychological needs at different stages of life-span:

- **Infancy:** This period extends from birth to 18 months of age. This is called the age of trust vs mistrust. The infant who comes to the new environment, from mother's womb needs only nourishment. If the child's caretaker anticipates and fulfills these needs consistently, the infant learns to trust others, and develops confidence. Unfulfillment of these needs enable the child to develop anxiety and rejection. If the infant fails to get needed support and care, it develops mistrust which affects the personality in later stages of life.
- **Toddler:** This stage ranges from 18 months to 3 years. By second year of life, the muscular and nervous systems have developed markedly and the child is eager to acquire new skills. The child moves around and examines its environment under the guidance of parents. Child starts developing independency in acquiring new tasks. Over protection and control on child can make him worthless and shameful of being capable of so little.

- **Preschooler:** This stage extends from 3 to 5 years. Once a sense of independence has been established, the child wants to tryout various possibilities. It is at this time the child's willingness to try new things is facilitated or inhibited. Identification of creative efforts and providing favorable direction will helps the child to take further initiative otherwise the child may develops feelings of guilt.
- **School age:** This period ranges from 5 to 12 years. During this period the child develops greater attention span, needs less sleep, and gains rapidly in strength; therefore, the child can expend much more effort in acquiring skills, and needs accomplishment, regardless of ability. The crisis faced during this period is industry vs inferiority.
  The child aims to develop a feeling of competence, rather than inability. The success in this endeavor leads to further industrious behavior, failure results in development of feelings of inferiority. Hence, the caretakers should guide the child to take up appropriate tasks.
- **Adolescence:** This is a period of transition from childhood to adulthood which extends from 12 to 20 years. During this period the individual attains puberty leading to many physical and psychological changes. These changes have enormous implications for the individual's sexual, social, emotional and vocational life; that is why Stanley Hall has rightly described this period as a '*period of storm and stress*'.
  These changes make the individual to find an identity, which means developing an understanding of self, the goals one wishes to achieve and the work/occupation role. The individual craves for encouragement and support of caretakers and peer groups. If he is successful he will develop a sense of self or identity, otherwise he will suffer from role confusion/ identity confusion.
- **Early adulthood:** This stage extends from 20 to 30 years. As an adult, the individual takes a firmer place in society, usually holding a job, contributing to community and maintaining a family and care of offspring. These new responsibilities can create tensions and frustrations, and one solution involves is, an intimate relationship with family. This situation leads to a crisis called intimacy v/s isolation.

If these problems are solved effectively by the love, affection and support of family the individual leads a normal life, otherwise he will develop a feeling of alienation and isolation which in turn affects his personality negatively.

- **Late adulthood:** This period ranges from 30 to 65 years. It is otherwise called middle age. During this stage of life, the crisis encountered is generativity vs stagnation. This requires expanding one's interests beyond oneself to include the next generation. The positive solution to the crisis lies not only in giving birth to children, but also in working, teaching and caring for the young, in the products and ideas of the culture, and in a more general belief in the species.
  This response reflects a desire for well-being of the humanity rather than selfishness. If this goal is not achieved the individual will be disappointed and experience a feeling of stagnation.
- **Old age:** This stage is the extension after 65 years till death. By this age people's goals and abilities have become more limited. In this stage an individual goes in flashback to find meaning in memories and explore tasks he had completed at a particular stage of life. If an individual found meaning in certain goals, or even in suffering, then the crisis has been satisfactorily resolved. If not, the person experiences dissatisfaction, and the prospect of death brings despair. The declining physical health conditions, decreased income, death of spouse, etc. will still more worsen these feelings.

PSYCHOLOGICAL NEEDS OF VULNERABLE POPULATION

Individuals are vulnerable when their physical security or health is at-risk. An individual may be vulnerable as a result of inadequate access to resources, inadequate protection from an external threat, and/or personal limitations in relation to the context in which he or she is living. All human beings require access to vital resources such as clean water, food, shelter, clothing, and sanitation. Not adequately meeting their basic mental, emotional or social development needs is an additional risk for individual.

Vulnerability may also be imposed on an individual by others through persecution and abuse based on gender, race, ethnic or political differences. Alternatively, vulnerability may spring from the individual due to personal limitations or weaknesses. Personal limitations that can cause vulnerability include:

- **Physical limitations:** Inadequate strength, size, health, capabilities.
- **Social marginality:** Inability to obtain necessary social protection, cooperation, assistance, or support.
- Inadequate knowledge or skills.
- **Mental/emotional disabilities:** Inability to function normally in a given social context.

Needs of children: In general, children are best cared for by their parents. Children need love, affection, good nutrition and good social environment for harmonious growth. It is responsibility of parents to monitor the growth and development of a child since birth itself. Nation development depends on the growth and development of children. In recent era, changes and implementation of many law related to children brought a remarkable change in the life of children. Still, certain root problems like child abuse, trafficking, child labor and lack of education deserve attention for uplifting the status of children in society.

Needs of elderly: Individuals experienced many changes as they age. Physical changes occur in virtually every body system. Psychological, there may be age-related cognitive changes in memory, judgment, attention and concentration, etc. individual in old age need more attention in terms of love, sympathy, involvement in decision making, social interactions to beat isolation and survive the life without any psychological problems. Elderly have very specific needs as compare to adolescent and adult. Sleep problem is very common in old age people. In terms of food, elderly need light food that can be easily digestible and excrete out.

Needs of women: Women are specific group of our society. We cannot imagine the completeness of the world without women and their contribution in society. Women deserve recognition and respect from other individual in the society. In present era, more empowerment and opportunities for women made them independent in their role. Still, women need more attention in terms of meeting different need related to education, food, respect and recognition in few of societies.

Psychology during illness: The way in which an individual is affected psychologically is dependent on many factors. Some of these include the nature of the illness itself, its severity and the treatment involved. Other factors impacting an individuals' ability to cope have to do with their personality, circumstances of their life prior to the illness and the level of social support that they have access to. Regardless of these factors, all individuals must go through various stages as they attempt to adjust and cope to the realities of their chronic condition.

Initially there may be shock, denial and disbelief that something is going wrong. The persistence of symptoms however makes it difficult to ignore. Resistance to the real changes occurring in the body cause a person to push themselves beyond what their body can do, creating more exhaustion and 'crashing' while they attempt to recover. Feelings of anxiety and fear occur in response to the uncertainty of the future; and the possible loss of goals unrealized contributes to sadness, depression and grief.

NURSING IMPLICATIONS OF GROWTH AND DEVELOPMENT

The nurse is involved in assessing development at each stage, and in providing anticipatory guidance to families to foster optimal development.

- **To understand behavior of patient:** Nurses work in a setting where they are required to interact with other professionals in an effort to bring the best quality care for their patients. They need to fully understand how other people behave and act in certain situations—this is where psychology comes into play.
- **To manage patient:** In managing patients with different illnesses, both nurses and psychologists not only work in understanding the physical pain associated, but also change their thought and attitudes to improve well-being.
- **To assess patient in healthcare setting:** When assessing a patient's condition, nurses also consider how patient's respond to their illness. Some patients are optimistic and easily cope with their illness, while others have a negative reaction where they become angry and stubborn. Nurses may find it very difficult to handle such patients and need to include them as part of their evaluation of the patient.
- **To communicate with patient:** With the help of psychology, nurses will know how to interact with their patients based on different factors such as gender and age. For instance, young patients may be more afraid than adults. They may have difficulties in understanding their illness. A nurse can apply

his knowledge of child development and psychology and relate to the young patients in a way their apprehensions are alleviated. Thus, psychology can help improve the nurse and patient relationship. As a result, patients can openly interact and communicate with them and inform them about their specific needs.

- **To develop rapport with patient**: With the help of psychological knowledge, nurses are able to get the trust of their patients. This makes the patients more responsive with the instructions they are given. Sometimes, they even take a positive role in their own wellness.

Suggested Reading

- Baltes PB. Theoretical Propositions of Life-span Developmental Psychology: On the Dynamics Between Growth and Decline. Developmental Psychology. 1987;23(5):611-26.
- Barkway P. Psychology for Health Professionals. 2nd ed. Australia: Elsevier. pp 26-48.
- Berman A, Snyder SJ. Kozier and Erb's Fundamental of Nursing. 9th ed. New Jersey: Pearson Education. pp 352-78.
- Bhatia BD, Craig M. Elements of Psychology and Mental Hygiene for Nurses in India. 2nd ed. Hyderabad: Universities Press. pp 317-25.
- Feldman RS. Essentials of Understanding Psychology. 11th ed. New York: McGraw-Hill Education. pp 327-60.
- Kyle T, Carman S. Essentials of Pediatric Nursing. 2nd ed. Philadelphia: Wolters Kluwer Health. p 71.
- Morgan CT, King RA, Schopler J. Introduction to Psychology. 7th ed. New Delhi: Tata McGraw Hill Publishing Company. pp 415-75.
- Pedersen DD. Psych Notes: A Clinical Pocket Guide. Philadelphia: FA Davis Company. pp 7-9.
- Potter PA, Perry AG. Fundamental of Nursing. 8th ed. St. Louis, Missouri: Elsevier. pp 130-75.
- Snyder CR, Lopez SJ. Oxford Handbook of Positive Psychology. 2nd ed. New York: Oxford University Press. pp 117-30.
- Sreevani R. Psychology for Nurses. 1st ed. New Delhi: Jaypee Brothers Medical Publishers. pp. 188-95.
- Williams PG, Holmbeck GN. Adolescents Health Psychology. Journal of Consulting and Clinical Psychology. 2002;70(3):828-42.

REVIEW QUESTIONS

SHORT-ESSAY TYPE QUESTIONS

1. Define growth and development. Explain the difference between growth and development.
2. Explain Freud's theory of psychosexual development.
3. Explain the principles of growth and development.
4. Explain the various factors which influence growth and development.

MULTIPLE CHOICE QUESTIONS

1. At what time of life does Erikson stage Industry vs. Inferiority occur?
   a. Old age
   b. Adolescence
   c. Infancy
   d. School age
2. Which of these are associated with insecurely attached infants in later life?
   a. Less competent
   b. Has less mature friends
   c. Less socially skilled
   d. All of the above
3. If a young adult sees stealing as wrong because of the harm it brings to someone, which of Kolberg's stages are they displaying?
   a. Punishment and obedience orientation
   b. Good boy good girl orientation
   c. Legalistic orientation
   d. Social order orientation
4. Which of these is a misconception about heredity?
   a. Heredity means that a person will not change.
   b. It is a waste of effort to try to influence a trait that has a strong heredity component.
   c. If the heritability of a trait is high, it shows that society has had little influence on the trait.
   d. All of the above
5. According to Erikson's eight stages of psychosocial development, during which age does the psychological stage of trust vs. mistrust develop?

a. Early childhood
b. Infancy
c. Adolescence
d. Adulthood

6. Which of the following is a way to measure activity level in an infant?
   a. How often they smile?
   b. How much they sleep?
   c. How much they want to be held?
   d. All of the above

7. Which of the following is NOT true for Growth?
   a. Growth is structural.
   b. Growth is quantitative.
   c. Growth is cellular.
   d. Growth is a lifelong process

8. Which indicates the change in the quality or character of a child?
   a. Growth
   b. Development
   c. Learning
   d. Environment

ANSWER KEY

1.	d	2.	d	3.	c	4.	d	5.	b	6.	b	7.	d
8.	b												

Mental Health and Mental Hygiene

Chapter 13

INTRODUCTION

Health and illness are defined according to the values of society to which a person belongs, when a person is able to adjust and adapt to his/her environment he/she is said to be healthy. A person with good mental health functions comfortably with society.

MENTAL HYGIENE

Mental hygiene is a science which deals with the process of attaining mental health and preserving mental health in the society. The term mental health is closely related with the term mental hygiene as the main objective of mental hygiene is to attain mental health. In other words, mental hygiene is a means of mental health. That is why we can say that mental hygiene is the means and mental health is the end.

Mental hygiene deals with those principles of living which would serve as a guide to human adjustments. It consists of those patterns of living which promote the development of wholesome and socially adequate personalities. These patterns of living help an individual to avoid conflict and to make better adjustment. So the focus of mental hygiene is on human adjustment.

Definition

'Mental hygiene is an endeavor to aid people to ward off trouble as well as to furnish ways of handling trouble in intelligent fashion when it cannot be warded off.' To him, these troubles may be illness, finances, social positions, sex, economic security, old age, inadequate shelter, etc. (Klien)

According to Rivillin mental hygiene refers to:

- The application of a body of hygiene information and technique.
- It is taken from the sciences of psychology, child psychology, education, sociology, psychiatry, medicine and biology.

- It cares for the purpose of the preservation and improvement of mental health of the individual and community.
- It is meant for prevention and cure of minor and major mental diseases and defects of mental, educational and social mal adjustment.

Mental hygiene consists of measures to reduce the incidence of mental illness through prevention and early treatment and to promote mental health. (Singh and Tiwari, 1971)

OBJECTIVES OF MENTAL HYGIENE

Mental hygiene is a science. The main objective of mental hygiene is to build up one's ego rather than tearing down another's ego. It tries to develop the power of tolerance and praise and discourages the habit of blaming others. Hence, we can say that the approach of mental hygiene is positive rather than negative.

The objectives of the mental hygiene can be summarized as shown below.

- **To help to realizes one's potentiality:** Every individual possess certain potentialities. Mental hygiene tries to help each individual to develop his/her potentialities.
- **To develop self-respect and respect for others:** Loss of self-respect is one of the factors for the great majorities of emotional disorders. A person who likes himself can like others and one who dislikes himself cannot like anybody. Hence, the main aim of mental hygiene is to help one to respect oneself.
- **To understand one's limitations and tolerate the limitations of others:** Mental hygiene helps one to understand his own limitations as well as to tolerate others' limitations.
- **To cause harmonious development:** Mental hygiene aims at the harmonious development of the physical mental and spiritual capacities of the individual so that he can adjust himself in the environment.
- **To create happiness:** Another objective of mental hygiene is to develop a positive attitude towards life so as to create a sense of happiness in a person who can live happily in this world.
- **To enable one to make effective adjustment:** Mental hygiene also prepares an individual for effective adjustment in all sphere of life and all situations such as in school, home, society work and also with self.

- **To enable one to know his or her self:** Many of us do not know our own self. We are not at all aware about our potentialities, weaknesses, limitations, etc. for which many individuals suffer from different types of confusion. Mental hygiene helps an individual to know himself.

FUNCTIONS OF MENTAL HYGIENE

Mental hygiene has four important functions. These are:

1. **Prevention or preventive:** The most important function of mental hygiene is to prevent mental health problems by developing some programs.
2. **Creative:** Another function of mental illness is to develop program like counseling, psychotherapy to treat an individual or a group or to treat a mental patient.
3. **Preservative:** Not all people are mentally ill; rather of them possess sound mental health. So the third function is to develop program through education for preserving mental health.
4. **Training:** Another function of mental hygiene is to train a set of personnel who can help the people with psychological problem by trying to understand their problems and then helping them to meet their needs.

To formulate general principles of mental hygiene is a really difficult task as there is a wide range of differences among the individuals. Some of the reasons for this are:

Human beings have multiple needs which grow in the course of development. These needs are contradictory in nature.

There is no single, also absolute standard to judge human behavior or action.

However, in spite of these difficulties, we can formulate some general principles. These are:

- **Adjustment in home:** Every child should develop such type of behavior at home so that he can adjust himself in any type of situation. Parents should take utmost care because the behavior patterns that develop in early childhood leave permanent impression on the child. Parents should try to develop the desirable traits in their children and develop competence, security, adequacy, self-esteem and discipline by catering to their basic needs.
- **Adjustment in school:** After home, school plays an important role in the development of personality. The school through its

various activities can go a long way in creating an environment for the children to preserve and develop their mental health.

- **Adjustment to society:** Man is a social animal and he has to adjust himself with the society. Without proper social interaction, harmonious development of personality cannot occur. Hence, parents, teacher and society must provide socially acceptable channels for the release of pent up emotional feeling so that the children and adolescents develop healthy personality.
- **Adjustment to work:** According to Freud, one is mentally healthy, if one can work successfully. School through its program, should develop the proper mental state towards work in child.

MENTAL HEALTH

Introduction

Mental health is how we think, feel and act as we cope with life. It also helps determine how we handle stress, relate to others and make choices. Like physical health, mental health is important at every stage of life, from childhood and adolescence through adulthood.

Everyone feels worried, anxious, sad or stressed sometimes. But with a mental illness, these feelings do not go away and are severe enough to interfere with your daily life. It can make it hard to meet and keep friends, hold a job or enjoy your life.

Mental health is a level of psychological well-being, or an absence of mental illness. It is the 'psychological state of someone who is functioning at a satisfactory level of emotional and behavioral adjustment'.

According to the *World Health Organization (WHO)*, mental health includes 'subjective well-being, perceived self-efficacy, autonomy, competence, intergenerational dependence, and self-actualization of one's intellectual and emotional potential, among others'.

Definition

Mental health is a positive state in which one is responsible, displays self-awareness, is self-directive and is reasonably worry-free and can cope with usual daily tensions.

Mental health is a state of emotional, psychological and social wellness evidenced by satisfying interpersonal relationships, effective behavior and coping, a positive self-concept and emotional stability.

'Mental health is a simultaneous success at working, loving and creating with the capacity for mature and flexible resolution of conflicts between instincts, conscience, important other people and reality'. (American Psychiatry Association, 1980)

'According to mental health is a dynamic state in which thought feeling and behavior that is age appropriate and congruent with the local and cultural norms is demonstrated'. (Robinson, 1983)

Other definitions refer to the ability to:

- Solve problems.
- Fulfill one's capacity for love and work.
- Cope with crises without assistance beyond the support of family or friends.
- Maintain a state of well-being by enjoying life, setting goals and realistic limits, and becoming independent, interdependent.
- It requires a balance between the body, mind and spirit and the environment in which the person lives (Fig. 13.1).

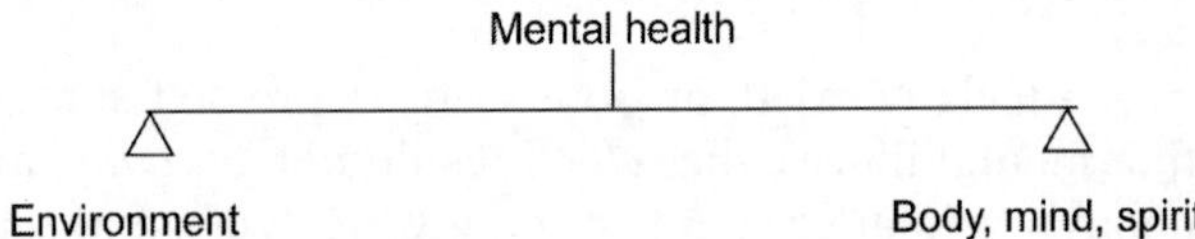

Mental health as balance between environment and body, mind and spirit

Fig. 13.1: Concept of mental health

CHARACTERISTICS OF MENTALLY HEALTHY PERSON

Mental health refers to our positive characteristics and overall psychological well-being. Mentally healthy people are known to deal with stress effectively by being able to bounce back from adversity. They are basically content people whose activities and relationships are meaningful.

Some characteristics of mentally and emotionally healthy people are outlined as follows:

- Maslow (1954), an eminent psychologist and writer, developed the following ideas about mentally healthy people:
  - **Self-acceptance:** They possess the ability to accept themselves, others and nature. They have positive self-concepts and relate well to people and their environment.

- **Make and maintain relations:** They are able to form close relationships with others. Kindness, patience and comparison are displayed for others.
- **Live in reality:** They perceive the world as it really is and people as they really are. Problem-solving occurs because these people are able to make decisions pertaining to reality rather than fantasy.
- **Enjoy life:** They are able to appreciate and enjoy life. Optimism prevails as they respond to people, places and things in daily encounter.
- **Independent in thought and actions:** They are independent or autonomous in thought and action and rely on personal standards of behavior and values. Such persons are able to face with reality and happiness, circumstances that would drive other people to self-destructive behavior.
- **Creative nature:** They are creative, utilizing a variety of approaches as they perform tasks or solve problems.
- **Respect others:** Their behavior is consistent as they appreciate and respect the rights of others, display a willingness to listen and learn from others and show severance for the uniqueness and difference in others.

• WC Menninger (of the Menninger Foundation) summarized emotional maturity as the:
  - Ability to deal constructively with reality.
  - Capacity to adopt change.
  - Relative freedom from symptoms produced by tensions and anxieties.
  - Capacity to find more satisfaction in giving than receiving.
  - Ability to relate to other people in a consistent manner with mutual satisfaction and helpfulness.
  - Capacity to redirect one's instinctive hostile energy into creative, constructive outlets.
  - Capacity to love.

• Jahoda (1958) has identified a list of six indicators that she suggests are a reflect of mental health:
  1. **A positive attitude toward self:** This includes an objective view of self, including knowledge and acceptance of strength and limitations. The individual feels a strong sense of personal identity and a security in the environment.
  2. **Growth development and the ability to achieve self-actualization:** This indicator correlates with whether the

individual achieves the tasks associated with each level of development. With success of achievement in each level the individual gains motivation for advancement to his or her highest potential.

3. **Integration:** The focus here is on maintaining an equilibrium or balance among various life processes. It includes the ability to adaptively respond to the environment and the development of a philosophy of life, both of which help the individual maintain anxiety at a manageable level in response to stressful situations.
4. **Autonomy:** This refers to the individual's ability to perform in an independent, self-directed manner. The individual makes choices and accepts responsibility for the outcomes.
5. **Perception of reality:** This includes perception of the environment without distortion, as well as the capacity for empathy and social sensitivity–a respect and concern for the wants and needs of others.
6. **Environmental mastery:** This suggests that the individual has achieved a satisfactory role within the group, society or environment. Also, suggests that he or she is able to strategize, make decisions, change, adjust and adapt according to the situation.

- Johnson (1997): Component of mental health includes:
  - Autonomy and independence
  - Maximizing one's potential
  - Tolerating life's uncertainties
  - Self-esteem
  - Reality orientation
  - Stress management
  - Mastering the environment.

WARNING SIGNS OF POOR MENTAL HEALTH

Symptoms of mental disorders vary depending on the type and severity of the condition. Some general symptoms that may suggest a mental disorder include:

In Younger Children

- Changes in school performance
- Poor grades despite strong efforts
- Excessive worrying or anxiety

- Hyperactivity
- Persistent nightmares
- Persistent disobedience and/or aggressive behavior
- Frequent temper tantrums.

In Older Children and Adolescents

- Inability to cope with daily problems and activities
- Changes in sleeping and/or eating habits
- Abuse of drugs and/or alcohol
- Excessive complaints of physical problems
- Intense fear of gaining weight
- Frequent outbursts of anger
- Skipping school frequently, stealing or damaging property
- Long-lasting negative mood, often along with poor appetite and thoughts of death.

In Adults

- Confused thinking
- Long-lasting sadness or irritability
- Extreme high and low in moods
- Excessive fear, worrying or anxiety
- Social withdrawal
- Strong feelings of anger
- Dramatic changes in eating or sleeping habits
- Delusions or hallucinations
- Increasing inability to cope with daily problems and activities
- Thoughts of suicide
- Denial of obvious problems
- Many unexplained physical problems
- Abuse of drugs and/or alcohol.

Enhancing Mental Health

By trying to analyze our motives and abilities, we can enhance our capacity to make active choices in our lives instead of passively accepting whatever happens. A few general suggestions have emerged from the experiences of therapist. These are:

- Accept your feelings
- Know your vulnerabilities
- Develop your talents and interests
- Become involved with other people
- Know when to seek help.

MENTAL ILLNESS

Mental illness occurs when a state of physical, mental, social and spiritual well-being is disturbed.

Mental illness means the maladapted and disordered psychological functioning of an individual. Thus mental illness brings about conditions of behavior which hinder adequate adjustment to life situations. The person who becomes the victim of mental illness is incapable of solving life's problems in a socially acceptable manner; his behavior will be abnormal.

Mental illness refers to an illness which manifests as abnormalities of personality, behavior, thought, mood, intellectual functions causing distress to self and society. This makes him/her dysfunctional in all or some areas of lives that is activities of daily living, covering personal, family, social and work.

Definition

'A clinically significant behavioral or psychological syndrome or pattern that occurs in an individual and that is associated with present distress (e.g. a painful symptoms) or disability (i.e. impairment in one or more important areas of functioning) or with a significantly increased risk of suffering death pain, disability or an important loss of freedom'. (American Psychiatric Association)

'Maladaptive responses to stressors from the internal and external environment, evidenced by thoughts, feelings and behaviors that are congruent with the local and cultural norms and interfere with the individual's social, occupational and physical functioning'.

(Townsend, 1996)

'Collectively to all diagnosable mental disorders (which) are health conditions that are characterized by alteration in thinking, mood or behavior (or some combination thereof) associated with distress and or impaired functioning.'

(Substance Abuse and Mental Health Administration, 1999)

Characteristics of Mental Illness

- Abnormal changes in one's thinking, feeling, memory, perception, and judgment resulting in the changes in talk and behavior.
- These changes cause distress and suffering to the individual or others around him.
- The abnormal changes and the consequent distress cause disturbance in day-to-day activities, work and relationship with important others.

Causes of Mental Illness

There is no single cause for mental illness. A long list of risk factors are there that may predispose an individual to mental illness. Some of the important risk factors are listed here:

- Biochemical changes in the brain
- Hereditary/genetic factors
- Changes in structure and functions of the brain (brain infections, brain tumor, nutritional deficiency, hemorrhage, accidents, etc.)
- Prenatal problems, i.e. antenatal preparation, accidents trauma, exposure to X-rays, etc.
- Personality and temperament development
- Lack of adequate love and care from the mother or separation of child from his/her mother
- Children from broken families
- Unable to cope with stress, tensions and frustration
- Loss of job
- Failure in business and examinations
- Death of life partner and loved one, etc.

Signs and Symptoms of Mental Illness

Mental illness may affect a person's physical health, mental functions, emotions and general health and overall behaviors.

- **Disturbances in physical functions:** Sleep, appetite and food intake, multiple physical complains, bowel and bladder movements, lack of interest in sexual activity.
- **Psychological symptoms:**
  - **Emotions:** Depressed, anxious, angry, sad, too happy, fearful, irritable, tearful with no reasons, etc.
  - **Talk and thinking:** May talk excessively and unnecessarily or may have a little or no talk. Talk may be irrelevant, incoherent and not understandable. May have strange ideas or false beliefs, delusion, preoccupation, etc.
  - **Perception:** Illusion, hallucinations, déjà vu and jamais vu, etc.
  - **Memory:** Poor memory power or frequent habit of forgetting.
  - **Intelligence and judgment:** Deterioration in intelligence power and decision-making capacity. Lose of reasoning skills and abilities.
  - **Level of consciousness:** Change in level of consciousness in some cases.
- **Changes in behavior:** Change in personal habits, social behavior, and personality, etc.

Misconceptions About Mental Illness (Table 13.1)

Mental illnesses are prevalent since the existing of human being. Belief about mental illness may be characterized in the form of superstition, ignorance and fear. Advancement of technology and mass media has dispelled these belief time-to-time. Some of common facts and misconceptions are discussed here.

Table 13.1: Misconceptions and facts about mental health

Misconceptions	Facts
• Mental illness is induced by black magic	• These illnesses have definite causes to occur
• Mental illness once acquired is lifelong	• Most of the illness can be controlled through effective treatment and family support. The only thing is that the person should take the medicine for a long period
• It is impossible to help someone with a mental illness	• Treatments do exist for this and caregivers can be assisted with the treatment
• Mental illness only affects adults in rich countries. Normal people will never become abnormal	• All are affected children, adolescence, adults, rich and poor
• We should just lock up the persons with mental illness	• Mental illness can be cured. They should be taken for treatment and treated in dignified manner
• All mentally ill patients show irrelevant behavior	• Very few patients show violent and irrelevant behavior
• Mentally ill people are not able to take decision	• Mentally ill people can take important decision after initial recovery
• Mental illness is contagious	• It is wrong to think that mental illness is contagious. It is not like TB, leprosy or other varieties of physical contagious disease. It cannot be spread by touching
• Marriage can cure mental illness	• Marriage cannot cure mental illness. To believe that marriage might be the cure for such illness is a wrong belief on the contrary, the patient's condition may turn to be worse than before. Marriage can become an additional stress. A patient who has recovered can get married and live a life like any other person
• Mental illnesses are of the same nature	• Not all mental illness is of the same nature

Strategies to Deal with Stigma and Prejudices

It can be done by:

- Making use of media of mass communication.
- Conducting public lecture, organizing mental health exhibitions and distributing pamphlets.
- Group discussion involving selected group like teachers, local leaders, traditional healers, etc.
- Encouraging the community to visit mental health centers.
- Advising the family to participate in treatment programs.
- Extending psychiatric services to general hospital.
- Demonstrating the usefulness of treatment.

Suggested Reading

- Mentak SD. Health and Psychiatric Nursing, 2nd ed. Makalu Publication, 2010; pp 1-7.
- Neupane KN, Shrestha R. Behavioural Science and Mental Health, 2nd ed. Makalu Publication. 2011; pp 141-54.
- Rawlins PR, Williams RS et al. Mental Health-Psychiatric Nursing, 3rd ed. Mosby: USA. 1993; pp 17-37.
- Shives RL. Psychiatric Mental Health Nursing, 2nd ed. JB Lippincott: Philadelphia. 1990; pp 1-6.
- Sreevani R. A Guide to Mental Health and Psychiatric Nursing, 3rd ed. Jaypee Brothers Medical Publishers (P) Ltd.: New Delhi. 2013; pp 1-2.
- Sreevani R. Psychology for Nurses, 2nd ed. Jaypee Brothers Medical Publishers (P) Ltd.: New Delhi. 2013, pp 158-60.
- Videbeck LS. Psychiatric Mental Health Nursing. Lippincott; Philadelphia. 2001; pp 148-50.

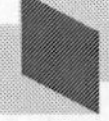

REVIEW QUESTIONS

SHORT-ESSAY TYPE QUESTIONS

1. Define mental hygiene. Discuss the objectives of mental hygiene.
2. Discuss various functions of mental hygiene.
3. Define mental health. Discuss the characteristics of a mentally healthy person.

MULTIPLE CHOICE QUESTIONS

1. Which of the following is an indicator of positive mental health?
   a. A positive attitude toward self
   b. Autonomy
   c. Environmental mastery
   d. All of the above
2. Which is not a cause of mental illness?
   a. Stress
   b. Genetic factors
   c. Biochemical changes in brain
   d. Getting good marks in exams
3. Which of the following is/are strategies to deal stigma or misconception about mental illness?
   a. Mass media
   b. Organizing camp
   c. Conducting public lectures
   d. All of the above
4. Which of the following is an early sign of poor mental health?
   a. Changes in sleep
   b. Disturbed appetite
   c. Disturbances in bowel habits
   d. All of the above
5. It is a science which deals with the process of attaining mental health and preserving mental health in the society.
   a. Mental health
   b. Mental hygiene
   c. Mental health nursing
   d. Psychology
6. The term 'Mental Hygiene' has been given to us by:
   a. CL Pierce
   b. CW Bears
   c. William James
   d. James D Page

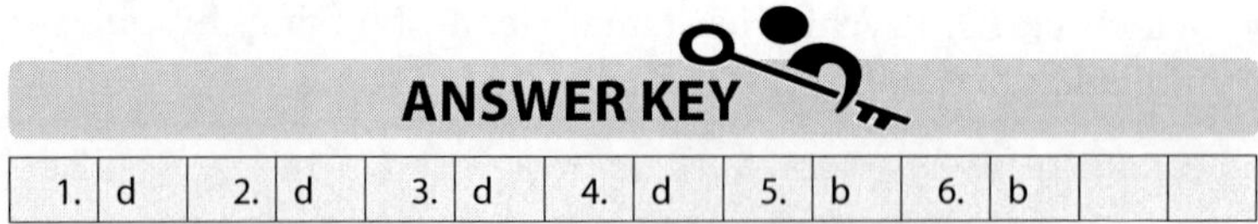

ANSWER KEY

1.	d	2.	d	3.	d	4.	d	5.	b	6.	b		

Chapter 14

Adjustment Psychology

DEFINITION

The behavioral process by which humans and other animals maintain equilibrium among or between their needs and the obstacles of their environments is so called adjustment psychology. A sequence of adjustment begins when a need is felt and ends when it is satisfied. Hungry people, e.g. are stimulated by their physiological state to seek food. When they eat, they reduce the stimulating condition that impelled them to activity, and they are thereby adjusted to this particular need.

In general, the adjustment process involves four parts: (1) a need or motive in the form of a strong persistent stimulus, (2) the thwarting or nonfulfillment of this need, (3) varied activity, or exploratory behavior accompanied by problem solving, and (4) some response that removes or at least reduces the initiating stimulus and completes the adjust. Researchers have interpreted adjustment from two important points of view.

1. **Adjustment as an achievement:** Adjustment as an achievement means how effectively an individual could perform his duties in different circumstances.
2. **Adjustment as a process:** Adjustment as a process is of major importance for psychologists, teachers and parents. To analyze the process we should study the development of an individual longitudinally from his birth onwards. The child, at the time of his birth is absolutely dependent on others for the satisfaction of his needs, but gradually with age he learns to control his needs. His adjustment largely depends on his interaction with the external environment in which he lives. When the child is born, the world for him is a big buzzing, blooming confusion. He cannot differentiate among the various objects of his environment but as he matures he comes to learn to articulate the details of his environment through the process of sensation, perception, and conception.

CONCEPT OF ADJUSTMENT

Adjustment is the relationship which comes to be established between the individual and the environment. Every individual plays certain position in his social relations. He is trained to play his role in such a way that his maximum needs will be fulfilled. So, he should play his role properly and get maximum satisfaction. If he does not play his role according to standards and training home environment received his needs may not be fulfilled and he may get frustrated.

TYPES OF ADJUSTMENT

- **Normal adjustment:** When a relationship between an individual and his environment is according to established norms then that relationship is considered as normal adjustment. A child who obey his parents, who is not unduly stubborn; who studies regularly and has neat habit is considered adjusted.
- **Abnormal adjustment:** Abnormal adjustment means problem behavior or popular speaking maladjustment. Maladjustment takes place when the relationship between an individual and his environment is not according to established standards or norms. A delinquent child adjusts with his environment but he is a maladjusted child because he is violating certain moral codes.

AREAS OF ADJUSTMENT IN NURSING

- **Social adjustment:** Every individual plays certain position in his social relations. He is trained to play his role in such a way that his maximum needs will be fulfilled. So, nurse should play his role properly and get maximum satisfaction. If she does not play his role according to standards and training, needs may not be fulfilled and she may get frustrated.
- **Emotional adjustment:** Nurse faces lots of emotions in her life, related to patients, her personal life, her occupational life, she has to adjust with all the emotions.
- **Occupational adjustment:** Nurse faces lots of problems at workplace. She faces many allegation and issues from patient and other healthcare members. For a beginner nurse, it is very difficult to adjust in strange hospital environment.

- **Physiological adjustment:** Social and cultural adjustments are similar to physiological adjustments. People strive to be comfortable in their surroundings and to have their psychological needs (such as love or affirmation) met through the social networks they inhabit. When needs arise, especially in new or changed surroundings, they impel interpersonal activity meant to satisfy those needs. In this way, people increase their familiarity and comfort with their environments, and they come to expect that their needs will be met in the future through their social networks. Ongoing difficulties in social and cultural adjustment may be accompanied by anxiety or depression.

CHARACTERISTICS OF A WELL-ADJUSTED PERSON

A well-adjusted person is able to make harmonious relationship with others in surrounding and able to deliver his role and responsibilities expected from him. Some of the characteristics of a well-adjusted person are given below:

- **Accept responsibility:** A well-adjusted person understands his position in the world and readily accepts the responsibilities that come with it.
- **Self-awareness:** He also knows his strengths and is constantly working towards improving on his weaknesses, which results in high self-esteem.
- **Self evaluation/introspection:** A well-adjusted person knows how to conduct realistic self-appraisals, taking account of where he has failed and where he has succeeded. This helps in the creation of realistic goals that help him reach his full potential.
- **Balance in life:** A well-adjusted person is self-driven, has a good work-life balance, and is motivated to achieve personal goals.
- **Commitment in relationships:** Another characteristic of a well-adjusted person is a commitment to relationships, career and business.
- **Responsible to work:** A well-adjusted person takes responsibilities seriously and does not commit to things he cannot complete.
- **Emotional stable:** He is emotionally stable and can control anger and other emotions well. Overall, the well-adjusted person is characterized as happy.
- **Face life challenges:** A well-adjusted person knows how to deal with life's challenges without compromising on the quality of his life.

- **Independent in thought and actions:** They are independent or autonomous in thought and action and rely on personal standards of behavior and values. Such persons are able to face with reality and happiness, circumstances that would drive other people to self- destructive behavior.
- **Make and maintain relations:** They are able to form close relationships with others. Kindness, patience and comparison are displayed for others.
- **Live in reality:** They perceive the world as it really is and people as they really are. Problem-solving occurs because these people are able to make decisions pertaining to reality rather than fantasy.
- **Enjoy life:** They are able to appreciate and enjoy life. Optimism prevails as they respond to people, places and things in daily encounter.

METHODS OF ADJUSTMENT

Usual method of overcoming blocks, reaching goals, satisfying motives, relieving frustrations and maintains equilibrium may be defined as *adjustment mechanism.* It helps in the following:

- It is a device by which an individual reduces his tensions or anxiety in order to adjust himself properly with the environment.
- It helps him to regain his mental health.
- It helps to solve his problems or to meet conflicting situations a child's uses certain self-adjustive, self-defensive approaches which may protect him from his frustrative situations. These are called defense mechanism.

CHARACTERISTICS OF ADJUSTMENT MECHANISM

Adjustment mechanism is almost used by all people. They are ideas which are inferred from the behavior of the individuals. All mechanisms are used to protect or enhance the person's self-esteem against dangers. They increase satisfaction and help in the process of adjustment if used within limit.

The danger is always within the person. He fears his own motives. The fear and danger are manifested in adjustment mechanism. The overall effect of adjustment mechanism is to cripple the individual's functioning and development through falsifying some aspects of his impulses so that he is deprived of accurate self-knowledge as a basis for action.

For example, a child is trained to sleep throughout the night without asking for milk. A child who plays his role successfully gets love and emotional security from his mother and he adjusts well to his home environment. On the other hand, if the child does not sleep properly and carries on his infantile role, he may get scolding and spanking from his mother. He may not be looked after properly and his mother's attitude may become indifferent and formal about him. Naturally the child may feel frustration. For example, once the child learns that while he is sleeping, his mother does not remain with him, his first reaction may be of frustration, then he may accommodate and later on, he may assimilate in the situation so completely that he may accept it as a part of life and he may not mind his mother's going out of his room while he is awake. The conscious and the rational method are known as direct method and unconscious method is known as indirect method.

WARNING SIGNS OF MALADJUSTMENT

- Conditions of tension and nervousness, deviations in feelings, acting and thinking are signs of maladjustment. The more serious the disorder, the more radical are the disturbances until a point is reached when the individual becomes almost incapable of adjusting to life. The maladjusted child may either show nervousness or may exhibit emotional over-reactions and deviations or may be emotionally immature.
- Living in fantasy or creating their own world is an another sign of maladjustment among adolescents.
- Regression to childish behavior.
- **Exhibitionistic or antisocial behavior:** The person may be suffering from psychosomatic disturbances.

SYMPTOMS OF MALADJUSTMENT

Many of the symptoms may be seen in maladjusted person but some of the important symptoms of maladjustment are given here:

- **Nervousness:** Nervousness in the person as exhibited by habitual biting and wetting of lips, nail biting, stammering, blushing, turning pale, constant restlessness, body rocking, nervous finger movements, frequent urination.
- **Undue anxiety:** The maladjusted person shows undue anxiety over mistakes, marked distress over failures, absent-mindedness, day-dreaming; he refuses to accept any recognition

or reward, evades responsibility, withdraws from anything that looks new or difficult, he has lack of concentration, is unusually sensitive to all annoyances is suitable to work when distracted and has emotional tone in argument and feel hurt when others disagree; he makes frequent efforts to gain attention of the teacher. Such are the emotional over-reactions and deviations.

- **Emotional instability:** The person is unable to work alone, and rely on his own judgment; becomes unusually self-conscious or overcritical of others, either too docile or too suggestive; such are his characteristic traits exhibiting his emotional in stability.
- **School maladjustment:** The person who cannot adjust himself in the school environment shows exhibitionistic behavior. He tends to tease, push and shove other pupils; he wants to be too funny or overconspicuous; he is either found bluffing, or refusing to accept any lack of personal knowledge; he agrees markedly with whatever the teacher says or does and shows exaggerated courtesy.
- **Antisocial behavior:** The maladjusted person has behavior disorders which are generally seen in his antisocial behavior. He is cruel to others, bullies them, uses obscene language, shows undue interest in sex, tells offensive stories, dislikes school work, resents authority, reacts badly to discipline, runs away from the class, and shows complete lack of interest in school work suddenly. He has psychosomatic disturbances also. When he is emotionally distressed, he begins to vomit or develops constipation and diarrhea or tends to overeat and shows other feeling disturbances.

FACTORS CAUSING MALADJUSTMENT

The five main causes of maladjusted behavior of adolescent are as follows:

1. **Family environment/issues:** The family as an institution has various functions to perform various causes, e.g. social, economic and psychological contribute immensely to maladjusted behavior in children.
2. **Social causes:** Gibbon says that the social problem of one generation is the psychological problem of the next generation. Children coming from homes that have been broken due to death, divorce, desertion, separation, etc. are often maladjusted in their behavior.

Such children feel insecure and become maladjusted. With the tremendous growth in population, it is extremely difficult for parents to provide even the basic necessities like food, clothing and shelter to their children. It invariably results in greater degree of frustration and hostility amongst them.

3. **Economic causes:** The occupational status of parents' problems of unemployment, poverty, and low economic status breed maladjustment amongst children.
4. **Psychological causes:** If parents are overpossessive highly authoritative, unrealistic in their expectations incompatible and abusive, this will have an adverse effect upon their children. When the psychological needs are not met, children get frustrated and develop problems like nail biting, fear of dark, lack of self-confidence.
5. **Personal causes:** The individuals who are physically, mentally and visually handicapped react abnormally to the situation. When they cannot score well academically compared to their peers, they develop an inferiority complex. Finally they isolate themselves from others and indulge in day-dreaming.

- **School-related causes:** When growing children do not find ways and means to channelize their energy in a purposeful manner in the school they exhibit in maladjusted behavior.
- **Teacher-related causes:** If the teacher is unfair, biased or not involved with the student it certainly affects the mental health of the children in the school.
- **Peer group-related causes:** Another important factor that disturbs the psychoequilibrium of students is an unhealthy relationship with their peer group.

Suggested Reading

- Aggarwal JC. Psychology of Learning and Development. Shipra Publishers: Delhi. 2007, pp 67-8.
- Bhatia MS, Craig M. Our Mental or Adjustment Mechanisms. Orient Longmann Publishers: New Delhi. 1968, pp 221-34.
- Mahmoudi A. 'Emotional Maturity and Adjustment Level of College Students. Education Research Journal. 2012;2(1):18-9.
- Walter Katkovsky, Gorlow L. The Psychology of Adjustment: Current Concepts and Application. New York: McGraw Hill Book Company, 1970.

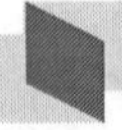

REVIEW QUESTIONS

SHORT-ESSAY TYPE QUESTIONS

1. Define adjustment. Explain concept of adjustment and maladjustment.
2. Discuss characteristics of a well-adjusted person.
3. Explain factors causing maladjustment and discuss warning symptoms of maladjustment.

MULTIPLE CHOICE QUESTIONS

1. Which of the following does not explain the true nature of adjustment?
   a. Adjustment is the process by means of which the individual attempts to maintain a level of physiological and psychological equilibrium.
   b. Only in death does the individual cease to adjust.
   c. Adjustment is an individual's behavior pattern directed towards tension-reduction.
   d. Adjustment is an attempt on the part of the individual to maintain harmonious relationship between himself and the environment.
2. The view that 'adjustment differs from maladjustment in degree rather than in kind' is psychologically:
   a. Correct
   b. Incorrect
   c. Correct sometimes
   d. Incorrect in certain situation
3. Which may not be a symptom of maladjustment?
   a. Nail biting
   b. Daydreaming
   c. Selfishness
   d. Excessive reading for vicarious excitement
4. Inadequate behavior pattern of the individual by means of which he attempts to adjust or satisfy his needs is known as:
   a. Defence mechanism
   b. Adjustment mechanism
   c. Maladjustment
   d. Withdrawal mechanism

5. The habit of smoking in students cannot be the result of:
   a. Modelling
   b. Inoculation
   c. Cigarete advertising
   d. Peer pressure
6. The word 'Adjustment' is biological in origin. It actually means:
   a. Survival
   b. Life
   c. Adaptation
   d. None of these
7. The most fundamental characteristic of good adjustments is:
   a. A sincere interest in people.
   b. A sound and wholesome system of motives and goals.
   c. A high degree of acceptance of one's environment.
   d. Keen insight
8. A well adjusted person should not have:
   a. Good health
   b. Happiness at work
   c. Unrealistic thinking
   d. Emotional center

ANSWER KEY

1.	b	2.	a	3.	c	4.	b	5.	b	6.	c	7.	b
8.	a												

Guidance and Counseling

Chapter 15

INTRODUCTION

Human life in this complex modern society is affected by a number of interacting factors. Personal and other problems have become part and parcel of life which affects every individual to some extent in his day-to-day life. The capabilities to solve personal, social, vocational and moral problems varies from individual-to-individual and sometime they require some assistance to overcome these problems from their grandparents, parents, other relatives and professional guidance and counseling service providers.

Similarly, any school or college of nursing is a miniature of this complex society where students from different backgrounds, cultures, and regions study and live together. A student can face a number of problems in campus as well as in out of campus life for which he seeks advice from his teachers or family members. Counseling explores the possible solutions for a problem situation and it depends on the person which solution he or she has to adopt. Nursing students as well as any other students may have a number of doubts, quires and problems related with their future, carrier, academic difficulties, learning difficulties and employment for which they need guidance from their teachers, who has to show them the right path so that they can succeed in their life as per their potential.

GUIDANCE

Meaning and Definition

Guidance is a broad concept which includes counseling in it, in other words counseling is a specialized and individualized part of guidance services. Thus, all counseling is guidance but all guidance is not counseling.

Some psychologists and educationists have defined guidance as following:

'Guidance is that aspect of educational program which is concerned especially with helping the pupil to become adjust in his present situation and to plan their future as per his interest, abilities and social needs.' (Erickson)

'Guidance is an assistance made available by a competent counselor to an individual of any age to help him to direct his own life, develop his own point of view, make his own decision and carry his own burden.' (Crow and Crow)

Types of Guidance

Every individual has limited capacity and sometimes they need assistance of a competent person to show them right path in a given situation, accordingly, the guidance may be of various types some of which are as following:

- **Educational guidance:** Educational guidance is provided to a student to assist him in selection of right educational stream, overcome academic problems, learning difficulties and motivate her to pursue right education path according to his interest, strength or potential.
- **Vocational guidance:** It is a type of carrier guidance in which students are assisted in the selection of right vocational carrier, employment and carrier opportunities, future scope and carrier growth by providing them related information so that student can make decision according to his resources and capabilities.
- **Social guidance:** Man is a social animal, for better adjustment in the society sometime, he may require assistance. Social guidance assist an individual to live with his full capacitates in the social environment, confirm to the social norms, develop healthy and positive social relationship, and regulate his social behavior and attitude so that, he can better adjust within and outside the school and college campus.
- **Personal guidance:** Personal guidance is provided to an individual student to overcome his personal problems and help him to better adjust with the school or college environment.

Needs of Guidance

- To assist an individual to solve a problem situation
- To satisfy educational, vocational and personal needs of a person
- To help an individual to adjust in a new environment

- To help an individual to select a course of study or professional course
- To help a person to select a job opportunity or employment.

COUNSELING

Meaning and Definition

Counseling involves more precision and depth in its approach as compared to guidance.

'Counseling is a personal and dynamic relationship between two individuals—an older, more experienced and wiser (counselor) and a younger, less wise (counselee). The latter has a problem for which he seeks the help of the former. The two work together so that the problem may be more clearly defined and the counselee may be helped to a self-determined solution'. (Wren, 1962)

'Counseling is the helping relationship that includes some one seeking help, someone willing to give help, who is capable or trained to help, in a setting that permits help to be given and received.' (Cormier and Hackney, 1987)

The definitions as stated above encompass the following elements of counseling.

- Counseling is a type of assistance which is received by a person who is in need of it.
- Counseling involves relationship between two persons, one who is overwhelmed with problem is at one end (counselee) and the other who assist the person to overcome the problem is a counselor at other end.
- Counseling helps an individual to develop objective view towards his problem situation.
- Professional counseling is never given; it is always taken by a person who is in need of it.
- Counseling does not mean solving the problems of others.
- Counseling is a personalized process, which depends upon the dynamics of interpersonal relationship.
- Counseling changes attitudes and behaviors of a person and makes him more confidants in dealing with a particular problem.

Counseling can be provided by an elder family member or relatives (*informal counseling*), as a part of professional work of some persons like nurses, social workers (*nonspecialist counseling*), and by a fully-trained person known as counselor who has obtained master's or PhD degree in psychology or guidance and counseling (*professional counseling*).

DIFFERENCES BETWEEN GUIDANCE AND COUNSELING

Table 15.1 depicts the differences between guidance and counseling.

Table 15.1: Differences between guidance and counseling

Counseling	Guidance
It helps with considering all sides of a potential choice even before the choice is made	Guidance is the process that is put in place at a time a choice is to be made
Counseling strictly observes the ethical principle of confidentiality	Guidance may or may not focus on confidentiality issue
It is individualized, specialized process with high level of precision and depth	It is a broad and comprehensive process
Counseling is a part of guidance, not all of it	Guidance is a term which is broader than counseling and which includes counseling as one of its concept
Counseling is more focused on social, personal and emotional problems of a person	Guidance mainly focus on educational and vocational problem of a person
Counseling is usually given for the abnormal behavior	Usually guidance is given to normal individual
It is always personal	It can be personal or impersonal
Changes are brought about in the feeling and emotions of the individual	Changes are brought in educational and vocational preferences of the individual

PRINCIPLES OF THE COUNSELING

- **Human dignity:** Every individual is different and represent personal values, traditions. Maintaining human dignity and accepting individual differences is primary concern of counseling process; counselee should not be made to feel inferior and subject to disrespectful behavior.
- **Hold personal values:** Counselor should be aware of his personal values and beliefs and should not impose the same on the counselee. The things the counselor may view as unimportant may be of paramount importance to the counselee. By keeping the personal values on hold the counselor can show empathy to the counselee.

- **Assist the client to make decision:** Counselor is not supposed to make decision for the client but he has to develop an objective view towards the problem situation with the help of client and explore the available alternatives for a given problem situation and assist the counselee to choose one as per his strength and willingness. It is strongly dedicated to self-direction and self-realization of the client or the student.
- **Nonjudgmental:** Be nonjudgmental, as a counselor you are not a judge.
- **Confidentiality and privacy:** Maintaining confidentiality and privacy is one of the important and ethical principle of professional counseling.
- **Voluntary:** Professional counseling is never given but it is always voluntarily sought by an individual who is in need of it.
- **Relationship:** Relationship of trust and confidence between counselee and counselor is of paramount importance upon which all the success of counseling process depends.
- The client's family members and significant others must be included in counseling process.

STEPS IN THE COUNSELING PROCESS

Counseling is a systemic process which passes through certain steps in order to achieve the success in counseling. These steps may be different depending on the counseling approaches used by the counselor in a particular session.

- **Establish trustworthy relationship:** Effectiveness of the counseling depend on the trust and warmth in the relationship between counselee and counselor. Establish a safe, physically comfortable, and calm environment with a feeling of warmth and acceptance towards counselee. Introduce yourself to the counselee and show acceptance and warmth in your conversation as the process of counseling advances. Respect and accept the individuality and uniqueness of the client, listen attentively, always address the counselee by his name, observe verbal and nonverbal communication and use of some common social skills are some important techniques to build rapport with the counselee.
- **Assessment:** This is the step in which counselee or counselees explore their feelings, problems and concerned area. Counselor encourages the counselee to express his personal view points

toward the problem situation and the emotional upset he is experiencing due to that problem situation, help the person put their concern into words. The role of the counselor in this phase is to develop an objective outlook of the problem so that possible interventions can be generated. Several specific skills are required for effective assessment which is as following:

- Active listening: find out the client's agenda
- Paraphrase, summarize, reflect, interpret
- Focus on feelings, not events
- Observations, enquiry
- Making associations among facts
- Making educated guesses
- Systematic and prompt recording of information.

- **Setting goals:** Counselor and counselee work together to set immediate and ultimate goals which are derived from the data, collected in assessment phase. Problem statements are transformed into goal statements. It requires the skills of drawing inference and differentiation from the collected data to set realistic goals for counselee.
- **Intervention:** Possible approaches to goal achievement are explored. The counsellor assists the counselee to choose one way towards goal according to his capacity and willingness. Develop a detailed plan to implement the intervention.
- **Termination and follow up:** Counselor summarizes what has occurred, clarify, and get verification from the counselee. Termination of the counseling session is done without destroying the accomplishments gained and with due sensitivity. Counselor may plan to get feedback and follow up appointment with counselee at regular interval if required.

TYPES OF COUNSELING APPROACH

Most of the available literature on guidance and counseling has described three types of counseling approach which are as following:

1. **Directive counseling or counselor centered or clinical counseling:** EG Williamson termed the directive counseling as clinical method. This approach is also known as authoritarian or psychoanalytic approach of counseling. As the name suggests that the counselor plays more active role and directs the process without violating the principles of counseling. He

assists the counselee in making decision and finding solutions to the problem. The main advantages of the approach are that it is economical in time and emphasizes the problem not the individual so that the counselor can see the counselee more objectively. Disadvantage of this approach is that the counselee becomes overdependent on the counselor.

2. **Nondirective counseling approach:** Carl Roger is the leading exponent of this counselee-centered humanistic approach of counseling. Here, the role of counselor is relatively passive and the client has to take the responsibility of exploring his problem situation, the counselor is neither agree nor disagree with the client but shows friendliness, and receptive attitude. In the beginning of the process counselor defines his limitations of the responsibilities and encourages the client to explore everything which is causing trouble to him. This approach put due emphasis on the individual and his potentials not on the problem.
3. **Eclectic approach of counseling:** Eclectic approach is the combination of the directive and nondirective approach of the counseling-based belief that counselor should be competent to use all available methods or resources. This approach suggests that the counselor should first take into consideration the personality, age, sex of the client as well as the type of problem; thereafter he should determine appropriate approach for counseling in that particular situation. The role of counselor is to plan and carry out the treatment of counseling and the responsibility of developing insight into the problem and making final decision rest on the counselee.

SKILLS/TECHNIQUES REQUIRED FOR EFFECTIVE COUNSELING

Counseling requires certain skills on the part of the counselor to effectively counsel the client by exploring the problem situation and suggesting alternatives for the same.

- **Active listening:** Easy to describe but difficult to practice it is the skill of listening to the client actively, attentively while maintaining eye to contact with the client and at the same time, observing the nonverbal behavior shown by the client. The technique of active listening includes:
  - Maintaining good eye-to-eye contact with client
  - Have open posture

  - Saying 'carry on' 'huhuu' 'nodding the head to agree with the client's statements' to encourage the client to speak more
  - Do not make any interruption in between when the client is talking
  - Ask questions whenever necessary to facilitate conversation.
- **Reflecting:** The counselor refers back the questions, feelings and any other important statements to the client so that, he can assume that the counselor understands what he intends to understand him.
- **Focusing:** Spotlighting the any idea or even a single word which seems to be significant for a given problem situation.
- **Summarizing and paraphrasing:** It is the brief restatement and rewording in own words of the main points what the client has communicated to the counselor to clarify the meaning of message so that the client can assume that the counselor has got the crux of his problem as well as the counselor becomes sure that he has understood what the counselee intends to communicate him.
- **Empathy:** Empathy is a skill of putting yourself into the shoe of other, means to think and feel a particular situation from the client's frame of reference. Empathy may be communicated verbally, nonverbally or by a mixture of both.
- **No scope for nontherapeutic technique use:** Giving reassurance, rejecting, giving advice, defending, using denial are some of the nontherapeutic communication techniques which the counselor should avoid during counseling.

PREREQUISITES OF COUNSELING

The preparation of the counselor can be divided into two categories: i. personal preparation and ii. preparation of the physical settings.

Personal Preparation

Self-awareness: Counselor should be aware of self prejudice, biases, feelings, value, motivation, personal strength and weakness. He should not have influence of these factors on the counseling process.

- **Physical appearance and health:** The physical appearance of counselor is also very important for success in counseling. He should have good physical appearance with proper gestures and postures. He should be physically fit.

- **Psychological health:** Good state of psychological health is required to be a good counselor. A counselor should be mentally healthy in all the aspects, aware of one's limitation, flexibility and adaptability should be there in his behavior.
- **Sensitivity:** A person who is aware of resources, limitation and vulnerability of other persons as well as is keenly perceptive to other person's feeling and needs is considered to have sensitivity.
- **Open mindness:** Counselor should prepare himself to accept the ideas or information openly without imposing any judgment and influence of his personal values.
- **Trustworthiness:** A counselor should be reliable, honest and maintain confidentiality of the information.

Physical Preparation

- The environment should be calm, quite, comfortable, soothing and esthetic. There should not be distracting stimuli which can disturb the process of counseling (switch off mobile phones, cut off the phone lines).
- There should not be a table (desk) between counselor and counselee as it can create barrier in the development of trustworthy and close relationship. If require, a desk can be placed at the side of the counselor to place tissue paper.
- The distance of sitting between counselor and counselee can have significant effect in the development of rapport. The distance should not be so close and so far but it should be maintained at the comfort level of the counselee which is determined by some variables such as cultural background, gender, age, etc. Distance of thirty to thirty nine inches has been found to be the average range of comfort between counselor and client of both genders *(Haase, 1970)*.
- The chairs for counselor and the counselee should be placed at right angle as it facilitates the counselee to either look at the counselor or straight ahead.
- Place 'Do Not Disturb sign', on the door to prevent others from entering when the counseling for one client is on progress.
- Assure auditory and visual privacy to the client as per the professional codes of ethics.

ORGANIZATION OF COUNSELING SERVICES

As discussed above there is great need to have formal counseling services in the setting of nursing educational institutes. Although, presently there is no such provision of formal counseling services for students in nursing schools and colleges, class teachers and principal are involved in guidance and nonprofessional counseling of the students. Numbers of factors are involved behind non-availability of the professional counseling services that includes lack of resources in colleges of nursing, lack of commitment on the part of administrator and management. Here, we will discuss how comprehensive program of formal counseling services in a college of nursing can be established.

A guidance and counseling committee can be established for the planning and implementation of the program under the overall control of principal college of nursing. Lecturer, in psychiatric nursing with certification in guidance and counseling can be appointed as programs coordinator in the initial phase to chalk out the purposes and framework of the services, identify available resources, and physical facilities for the same. A detailed program structure can be chalked out as per the institutional needs.

PROBLEMS IN COUNSELING

- **Lack of knowledge on the part of counselor:** Lack of knowledge of the different area of interest may pose a difficulty for the counselor. A counselor who is not through with the process, tools and techniques and basic communication skills may not serve as an effective counselor. It requires provision of in-service education for the nursing faculty so that they can provide effective guidance and counseling services for the nursing students.
- **Personal values:** It is mandatory for the counselor that he should keep on hold his personal values and preferences while providing counseling to the students, but it is quite difficult to achieve a satisfactory hold on the personal values for most of the nursing faculty and they impose the same on the counselee hence jeopardizing the objectives of the counseling.
- **Lack of objectivity:** Involvement of the subjectivity in the counseling process by the counselor reduces its effectiveness.

- **Lack of physical facilities and other resources:** Most of the nursing colleges are lacking in separate physical facilities and provision of professional guidance counselor which leads to disorganized and ineffective delivery of the counseling services to the students.

NEED OF GUIDANCE AND COUNSELING SERVICES IN NURSING

- Nursing education as well as nursing profession is unique as compared to other educational and workplace settings. Because of this uniqueness of the nursing education and nursing profession, guidance and counseling services are required in nursing educational institutions and nurse's workplace. Let us discuss these important issues which demand for guidance and counseling services at colleges of nursing as well as workplace of nurses.
- **Long duty hours:** Nursing students are supposed to perform long duties in clinical areas as per their curriculum requirement. Initially the students may feel difficulty to adjust the changing scenarios of life may experience maladjustment with the situation.
- **Hostel life:** Since nursing students has to live in nursing hostel with other colleagues which make a small society within the campus. There may be a number of problems associated with hostel life ranging from mess problem to lack of sleep because of different preferences of personal study hours among roommates. These problems really make a student puzzled and she requires guidance and counseling to solve these problems.
- **Night duty:** Students have to do night duty which is 12 hours long thereafter they are supposed to attend morning classes. This change in sleep cycle may disturb a student and he may feel burned out.
- **Personal problems**: There may a number of personal problems among nursing students ranging from love affair, love failure (most common problem in bachelor students), difficulty in understanding the contents, chronic illness which may become pathologic if appropriate guidance and counseling is not available at proper time.
- **High pressure of study**: The curriculum is vast and put high pressure of study to the students to get good marks on the students.

- **Altered sex ratio**: Majority of the students is female and the entry of male is limited. Hence the male students may have adjustment problem with the female colleagues and also they may feel isolation throughout the course of study.
- **Family problems**: Students may have family problems which may affect their academic performance.
- **Dealing with life and death situation**: Nursing profession is based on the principle of caring of sick and well. In the clinical area students witnesses the death of patients and crying relatives. Young students are not mature enough to deal with these situations psychologically and may require guidance and counseling support.
- **Getting experience not fit for age:** Young immature students are exposed to certain experiences which is quite unexpected in young age, e.g. putting Foley's catheter, witnessing deliveries, observing major surgeries and so on. Some students cannot cope with the situation initially and are in need of guidance and counseling services.
- **Playing role as staff nurses:** In most of the private nursing institutions nursing students are misused as staff nurses. They are given the responsibilities in clinical areas for which their shoulders are quite young and immature.
- **Lack of provision of stipend:** In private colleges and schools of nursing students are not paid stipend which may cause dissatisfaction among them and may demotivate them to learn and work in clinical area.
- **Suicide:** Nursing students are more stressed with their academics along with other problem which sometime may push a student to commit suicide to get rid of educational problems. In the past there are number of cases of nursing students in India which emphasize the need of counseling services in college itself so that precious lives can be saved.

NEED AT NURSES' WORKPLACE SETTING

- **Personal problem:** As mentioned previously personal problems are part and parcel of day-to-day life of every nurse. Personal problems affect job performance and thereby the performances of healthcare organization.

- **Increasing healthcare costs:** Healthcare costs are continued to rise day-by-day with the increasing level of inflation. Hence, reducing lateness, absenteeism, lost time with the help of guidance and counseling services can save money for a health care organization. Reducing turnover can improve productivity and the bottom line.
- Vulnerability of nurses is higher for feeling stressed out in nursing due to:
  - They need to act as mother, home manager, teacher, and manage critical situations in the high pressure clinical setting.
  - Hostel type accommodation provided to nurses by employers leads to problems of adjustment to hostel and mess.
  - Long hours clinical (night duty/shift duty).
  - Workload higher (nurse-patient ratio).
  - General training (most of nurses) but specific settings of work.
  - Poor working conditions.
  - Increased expectations of patients (patients' bill of right).
- Unfair remunerations to nurses.
- Round the clock duty leads to disorganized life of a nurse.
- Difficulty in getting leaves sanctioned leading to problems in family life.
- Less qualified supervisors (no value to higher degrees).
- Promotions issues: Promotion on the basis of experience only, no value of higher qualifications.
- Inability to meet job demands, over workload, confrontation with authority, responsibility and accountability.
- Conflicts with superiors, subordinates and management and various family problems, health problems, career problems, alcohol or substance abuse.
- Emotional problems, family or marital difficulties, financial or legal situations, workplace stress.

Suggested Reading

- Anand SP. ABC's of Guidance in Education, 5th ed. Mahamaya Publication House. 2005; pp 94-104.
- Arthur JJ. Principles of Guidance, 5th ed. McGraw Hill Book Company Inc. 1951; pp 209-14.

- Bhatia KK. Principles of Guidance and Counselling. Kalyani Publishers: Ludhiana. 2002; pp 75-197.
- Cormier LS, Hackney H. The Professional Counsellor: A Process Guide to Helping. Prentice-Hall Inc. Englewood Cliffs, New Delhi, 1987.
- Gibson RL, Mitchell MH. Introduction to Counselling and Guidance, 6th ed. Prentice-Hall of India Pvt. Ltd: New Delhi. 2003; p 290.
- Kochhar SK. Guidance and Counselling in Colleges and Universities. Sterling Publishers Private Ltd. 1984; pp 161–96.
- Lalitha K. Mental Health and Psychiatric Nursing. An Indian Perspective. 1st ed. VMG Book House. 2007; pp 144-51.
- Porter T, Grady O. The Nurse Manager's Problem Solver. Mosby: Philadelphia. 1994; pp 121-2, 211-2.
- Sharma R. Guidance and Counselling, 3rd ed (Reprint). Subject Publications. 2002; pp 268-88.
- Townsend MC. Essentials of Psychiatric Mental Health Nursing. FA Davis Company: Philadelphia. 1999; pp 111-6.

REVIEW QUESTIONS

SHORT-ESSAY TYPE QUESTIONS

1. Define guidance and explain areas/types of guidance.
2. Define counseling and explain types of counseling.
3. Explain difference between guidance and counseling.
4. Explain the need of counseling in nursing profession.

MULTIPLE CHOICE QUESTIONS

1. Education psychology is oriented towards:
   a. The study of the peculiarities of individual children.
   b. The application of the principles and techniques of psychology to the solution of the problems of the class room.
   c. The formulation of hypothesis and theories relative to educations practice.
   d. The development on the part of the child of realistic goals and effective plans for their attainment.

2. Which is not correct about social development of the child?
   a. It is continuous process by means of which the child achieves social adequacy.
   b. It is an attempt by society on having the child internalize certain of its regulations, values and mores.
   c. It is individualization meaning, thereby, child's attempt to retain some of his individuality.
   d. It is child's attempt on not going against anything that prevails in the society.
3. Which program should be based upon understanding the needs and problems of the students, competence and interest of the guidance personnel?
   a. Guidance tools b. Guidance principles
   c. Guidance services d. Guidance techniques
4. Dr Luke attends to emotionally disturbed students. Which guidance service is being provided by Dr Luke?
   a. Inventory service b. Information service
   c. Placement service d. Counseling service
5. A person's career includes any significant events and experiences but in which areas has work psychology been able to make a contribution?
   a. Career choice b. Career counseling
   c. Mentoring d. All of the above
6. Counseling is a profession that aims to:
   a. Promote personal growth and productivity.
   b. Provide successful diagnosis in psychopathology.
   c. Ensure that clients are on the correct education.
   d. Solely address behavior.
7. It is an assistance made available by a competent counselor to an individual of any age to help him to direct his own life, develop his own point of view, make his own decision and carry his own burden.
   a. Guidance b. Counseling
   c. Mentorship d. Advise
8. It is a types of guidance which delivered for better adjustment in the society and to live an individual with his full capacitates in the social environment and confirm to the social norms.
   a. Career guidance b. Social guidance
   c. Personal guidance d. Vocational guidance

9. It is a personal and dynamic relationship between two individuals in which an older, more experienced and wiser person helps a younger, less wise individual.
   a. Guidance b. Counseling
   c. Advise d. Mentoring

10. It is a types of counseling in which counselor play a passive role and client has to take the responsibility of exploring his problem situation.
    a. Directive counseling
    b. Non-directive counseling
    c. Elective counseling
    d. Clinical counseling

11. It is a counseling technique in which counselor refers back the questions, feelings and any other important statements to the client to understand what client intended to say?
    a. Nodding b. Reflection
    c. Restating d. Focusing

ANSWER KEY

1.	b	2.	b	3.	c	4.	d	5.	d	6.	a	7.	a
8.	b	9.	b	10.	b	11.	b						

Psychological Assessment and Tests

Chapter 16

INTRODUCTION

Psychological assessment also known as psychological testing is the process through which psychologists try to understand a person through a sample of his behavior obtained under a structured environment. Parents, teachers, and employers have always informally used limited observations of a person's behavior as clues to broader performance capabilities. When the procedure is more formalized, as in observing a person's behavior in response to strictly defined conditions, we call it a test (Jensen, 1981).

TYPES OF PSYCHOLOGICAL TESTS

Psychological tests can be broadly classified into the following four types:

1. Clinical interview
2. Tests of intelligence
3. Tests for personality assessment
4. Behavioral assessment.

- **Clinical interview:** It is a basic tool in the hands of a clinician and is an essential part of any psychological assessment session. Often times in itself it can be adequate. Depending on the purpose of the interview it could be a 'screening interview', 'therapy intake interview', 'diagnostic interview' or 'case-history interview'. These interviews last for about an hour and are conducted in a clinician's office. At times interview is a prelude to a psychological testing session to socialize the client to the testing atmosphere, to clarify doubts and to set the client at-ease.
- **Tests of intelligence:** Psychologists have devised many different kinds of intelligence tests each corresponding to the theoretical conceptualization of intelligence. As each one's conceptualization and description of the concept of intelligence

differs, the tests devised to assess the same also vary. These varied tests can be grouped into different categories based on the conceptualized component of intelligence, material used to assess, manner of administration, activity expected from the subject, time given for performance, etc. A broad classification of intelligence tests is as follows:

- **Individual vs group tests of intelligence:** Individual tests are administered to only one person at a time, as they require individual instructions, intensive observation, laying out of materials and accurate timing of performance. They are often used in counseling and hospital settings. Group tests on the other hand are administered to multiple subjects simultaneously. They facilitate obtaining information from multiple subjects at the same time and hence save time, energy and are cost-effective. These tests are often used in educational or industrial settings.
- **Verbal, non-verbal and performance tests of intelligence:** Verbal tests use language or verbal material to assess intelligence. Though almost all tests require written or oral verbal instructions, verbal tests heavily use verbal material as they assess processes such as verbal reasoning, verbal comprehension, verbal memory, etc. In a country like India it is cumbersome to develop verbal tests as there are multiple languages and what is developed in one region may not be applicable in a different region. Non-verbal tests are paper and pencil tests such as figural analogies, odd man out, number series completion, pattern completion, etc. Performance tests on the other hand, require the subject to draw, manipulate or construct something, e.g. figure copying, block designs, puzzle type problems, picture completion, etc.
- **Tests of capacity vs tests of competence:** They are also known as power tests and speed tests respectively. Some tests are untimed and the subject is left free to perform in their own pace. These tests assess the capacity of the person as he is allowed to use all his potential without any restraint of time. Timed tests on the other hand test the competence of the individual to perform a certain act within the stipulated time and hence are called tests of competence.

- **General ability tests:** Ability tests attempt to assess the overall average level of performance in a broad range of mental capabilities. In contrast aptitude tests are specialized tests to predict performance of a particular kind. Achievement test intend to assess specific attainments following a course of study.

- **Tests for personality assessment:** Assessing complex psychological constructs is not an easy task. While discussing the difficulties in measurement of personality SK Mangal (1998) discusses three elements playing a role in assessment of any psychological variable. They are:
  1. **What we want to measure:** Personality is a complex and dynamic phenomenon. How best can we assess something which is abstract and ever changing? An essential and first step in the process of assessing personality is to objectively define the concept.
  2. **Deciding how to measure it:** Based on the requirement one would choose from one of the personality techniques.
  3. **Deciding on who should be allowed to do the assessment**: The person or the examiner who is doing the assessment to a great extent affects the process of assessment. He/she has to be extensively and intensively trained in understanding the theoretical background of not only what is being measured but also about the process of measurement and the process of developing the tools of measurement. He/she needs to be trained so that his/her own individual or subjective factors do not contaminate the process of measurement.

Techniques or methods used to assess the personality:

- Certain tests require direct observation of the subject's behavior by the examiner in the natural or standardized environment, i.e. rating scales.
- The examiner questions the subject to obtain a predetermined set of information and using this information tries to estimate the personality of the subject, i.e. questionnaires.
- The examiner questions the people who observe the subject on a regular basis such as parents, teachers, spouses and uses the information to estimate the personality of the subject, i.e. rating scales, semistructured interview.
- An ambiguous stimulus is provided to the subject and the reaction of the subject to this novel and ambiguous situation

is observed and rated by the examiner for the purposes of personality assessment, i.e. projective tests (thematic apperception test, Rorschach ink blot test).
- Use of physiological, hormonal and neurological reactions to indirectly assess the underlying psychological attribute, i.e. psychophysiological assessments.

PURPOSE OF PSYCHOLOGICAL TESTS

Psychological tests are an integral and very important component of psychologists' armamentarium. Some of the purposes of psychological tests are:
- To assess the current level of cognitive and overall intellectual functioning and try to estimate the deterioration in relation to the premorbid levels of functioning.
- To screen for psychopathology and to assess the nature and severity of the psychiatric illness.
- To supplement, confirm or challenge the impressions formed through less structured assessment methods.
- To aid in the differential diagnosis of persons with complexities in clinical presentation.
- In a therapy setting—to assess the need for therapy, suitability for a particular mode of treatment, to assess the strengths and weaknesses in a person in order to decide the focus of therapy.
- To assess or monitor the improvement in cognitive functions, changes in psychopathology and general levels of functioning as a result of psychological treatment.
- To assess the differences in pre and posttherapy performance as part of clinical research.

CHARACTERISTICS OF A GOOD PSYCHOLOGICAL TEST

With the growing number of psychological tests and procedures that are developed through varied research designs, one is expected to choose the most appropriate test for use. Knowledge on certain characteristics of the tests, such as their reliability and validity, is essential for choosing a test.
- **Validity:** A test is deemed valid if it measures what it is supposed to measure. In other words the test is said to have validity to the extent that useful inferences can be drawn from the scores. That is, a test has validity if a person's performance on the test can tell you something about his performance in

some other situation. Predictive validity is the accuracy with which a test scores or a combination of scores can estimate a person's performance on some criterion such as school or job performance.

- **Reliability:** A reliable test on repeated administration will yield same results. A test's reliability can be interpreted as a tests correlation with itself. There are a number of methods for determining a test's reliability. Simplest method of them all is split half reliability where the whole test is given to a large number of people. Then the whole test is split in half, e.g. odd-numbered and even-numbered items. Correlation is computed between these two sets of scores. From this coefficient, reliability of the whole test is computed.
  Reliability is essential but not sufficient condition for test validity. A valid test is almost always reliable but a reliable test need not be valid.
- **Norms:** Norms is the third good characteristic of psychological tests. Norms is a set of score obtained by a group of population for whom the test is made. Norms helps to interpret the individual score on a psychological test.
- **Practicality:** Practicality refers to use and convenience of a test for population. It consists of economy, cost, usability, and interpretation of a psychological test. Test should be simple to administer with clear instructions. Test result should be easy to interpret and understand to expert as well as to others.

USES OF PSYCHOLOGICAL TESTS

Psychological tests play a significant role in a wide variety of situations. Freeman in his extensively read book 'Theory and Practice of Psychological Testing', enlists the following uses of psychological tests.

In general

- Determination of general intelligence.
- Assess the nature and course of mental development in infants and young children.
- Assessment of personality traits.
- To assess the personality differences associated with age, sex, culture.
- To assess intellectual and personality attributes of gifted population, mentally ill.

In educational setting

- Tests of intelligence have been extensively used in educational setting for educational classification, selection and planning of special services.
- To screen children with learning disabilities and to assess the type and severity of disability.
- To provide educational and vocational guidance.

In clinics

- To derive a clinical diagnosis.
- Assessment of cognitive functions such as attention and memory.
- Assessment of personality and interpersonal relations.
- Assessment of neuropsychological functions in psychiatric and neurological illnesses.

In industries

- Selection and classification of personnel for placement in jobs.
- Assessment of aptitudes and educational achievement.

ROLE OF NURSE IN ADMINISTRATION OF PSYCHOLOGICAL TESTS

Unlike lay persons, who lack knowledge of psychological testing at the best and carry misconceptions and spread them at the worst, nurse has the advantage of knowledge on psychological testing. A nurse, regardless of place of work or designation, has the duty to allay misconception in her patients, colleagues and others around and spread awareness.

A nurse working in a clinical setting, especially in a hospital providing the services of a psychiatrist and a psychologist, has the following responsibilities:

- To be sensitive to signs of psychiatric illness, emotional disturbances, behavioral oddities, developmental delays in her patients. Like any other paraprofessional he/she can administer basic screening tools and record the findings as nurse's notes. He/she then can communicate the findings to the treating clinician and facilitate further referral procedures.
- Patients who are referred for psychological assessment often are anxious and worried about the process and implications of the psychological assessment. A nurse needs to have adequate knowledge on the types of psychological tests and the process of

psychological assessment to socialize the patient to the process. She also needs to alleviate the anxiety in the client by clarifying their misconceptions and reassuring that the purpose of the assessment is to help the patient.

- To prepare the patient for the assessment and keep the patient physically comfortable as well as mentally relaxed just before the testing.
- Occasionally testing can elicit distressing emotions in patients and it may continue after the testing session. A nurse may have to be vigilant to such signs and report to the clinician if required.
- Nurses, trained in and offering psychotherapy services, should liaison with psychologists and make use of psychological assessment to decide on the focus of therapy and to monitor the progress of therapy.
- Wherever possible and permissible nurses should obtain training in administration of tools for clinical and research purposes.

IMPLICATIONS OF PSYCHOLOGICAL TEST IN NURSING

In clinical setting

- Knowledge on psychological tools would come in handy for nurses working in community health programs for identifying and referring high-risk cases for mental health services.
- With the growing need for mental health service and efforts from the government to make such services available at grass root levels, it is only imperative that nursing profession would be called upon to provide services in screening, assessment, intervention of people with mental illness. Adequate knowledge in this area would be an asset for a nurse venturing out into the field.

In academic setting such as nursing college

- Use of psychological tools by nursing tutors for selection, classification and promotion purposes.
- Assessment facilities and counseling facilities to be provided to students who are disturbed due to academic or personal stressors.
- Impart awareness in general public on mental health and psychological assessment facilities present in the community as part of health educations campaigns.

A nurse working in a research institute or teaching research

- To keep abreast of the new tools available for assessment of psychosocial variables.
- To help the student researchers to choose the right tests with adequate levels of reliability and validity.
- To facilitate training in administering the tools that are open for use by nurses.

Suggested Reading

- Anastasi A. Psychological Testing, 5th ed. Macmillan: New York. 1982.
- Freeman and Frank S. Theory and Practice of Psychological Testing, 3rd ed. Oxford & IBH: Calcutta. 1962.
- Jensen AR. Straight Talk About Mental Tests. The Free Press: New York. 1981.
- Mangal SK. General Psychology. Sterling Publishers: New Delhi. 1998.

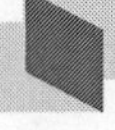

REVIEW QUESTIONS

SHORT-ESSAY TYPE QUESTIONS

1. Explain psychological tests and its uses.
2. Explain characteristics of a good psychological test.
3. Explain role of nurse in psychological tests.

MULTIPLE CHOICE QUESTIONS

1. Which of the following is NOT a characteristic of psychological test?
   a. Validity
   b. Reliability
   c. Usability
   d. Practicability
2. This is a type of psychological test which helps to test capacity of an individual to perform a particular task?
   a. Achievement test
   b. General ability test
   c. Competency test
   d. Aptitude test
3. It is a type of psychological test administered to a group of people to ascertain the information at a time?
   a. Individual test
   b. Group test
   c. Test of battery
   d. Intelligence test

4. Psychological test used for following purpose EXCEPT:
   a. Academic purpose
   b. To develop clinical diagnosis
   c. Screening mental disabilities
   d. To declare a person mental incompetent
5. A nurse help a psychologist to perform psychological test in following ways:
   a. Preparation of patient
   b. Training the patient to perform test
   c. Psychological assessment of patient
   d. All of the above
6. Which of following test used to test intelligence?
   a. Stanford-Binet test
   b. Rorschach inkblot test
   c. Thematic apperception test
   d. None of the above
7. What is Rorschach's projective test designed to measure?
   a. Unconscious intentions
   b. Dreams
   c. Conscious desire
   d. Brain size
8. Which of the following is not a projective technique?
   a. Word association test
   b. Thematic apperception test
   c. Sentence completion test
   d. Rorschach inkblot test
9. IQ test does not provide which of the following?
   a. High test-retest reliability
   b. Good predictor of behavior
   c. High internal consistency
   d. Good validity
10. Interview is the original method of:
    a. Selection
    b. Personality assessment
    c. Personality make up
    d. Attitude assessment

ANSWER KEY

1.	c	2.	c	3.	b	4.	d	5.	d	6.	a	7.	a
8.	a	9.	b	10.	b								

Index

Page numbers followed by *f* refer to figure and *t* refer to table, respectively.

B

C

D

E

F

N

R

T

U

V

W

Y